Sports Acupuncture

The Meridian Test and Its Applications

Sports Acupuncture

THE MERIDIAN TEST
AND ITS APPLICATIONS

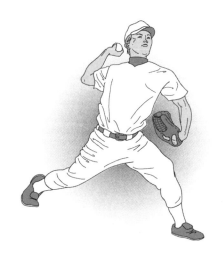

Mukaino Yoshito, M.D.

TRANSLATED BY STEPHEN BROWN

EASTLAND PRESS ▸ SEATTLE

Originally published in Japan in 2003 as *Sport Shinkyu Handbook* by Bunkodo Co., Ltd.
English translation rights arranged through Bunkodo Co., Ltd. with Eastland Press

English language edition ©2008 Mukaino Yoshito

Published by Eastland Press, Inc.
P.O. Box 99749
Seattle, WA 98139, USA
www.eastlandpress.com

ISBN: 978-0-939616-66-4
Library of Congress Control Number: 2008936740
Printed in the United States of America

2   4   6   8   10   9   7   5   3

Book design by Gary Niemeier

TABLE OF CONTENTS

PREFACE

....

UNTIL NOW, IN THE field of sports medicine, acupuncture has been perceived mostly as a modality for treating pain. Thus acupuncture has largely been relegated to the position of supplemental treatment for strains and injuries. Beyond its value in the rehabilitation of athletes, however, lately there has been a broader application of acupuncture aimed at improving conditioning and performance. The reputation of acupuncture as a very useful method for pre-game conditioning, as well as for recovery from fatigue, has been spreading among athletes and others involved in sports.

Be that as it may, there is a widespread impression that the traditional methodology of acupuncture is difficult to understand. Thus acupuncturists in Japan often rely on a simple methodology that matches empirical acupuncture points with specific symptoms. The truth is that, even for a single condition like low back pain, the effective points will vary for each athlete based on the specific characteristics of the sport, differences in athletic form, and differences in the alignment of the spine. For this reason, individualized treatment is required to attain the best results from acupuncture. Until now, however, there has been no easy-to-understand manual that explains how to provide individualized acupuncture treatment in the field of sports.

Around 1992, by coincidence, I found that one could quickly and easily determine the area of the body that needs treatment based on individual differences. This is done by incorporating the concept of acupuncture meridians and points in the observation of somatic responses to stress on the body during movement. Furthermore, the efficacy of this treatment is easily assessed. I developed this methodology through several years of trial and error and have called it the Meridian Test, or 'M-Test' for short. In 1995, I introduced the M-Test method at the FISU/CESU[1] conference at the Fukuoka Universiade.[2] Since that time, my colleagues and I have documented the results of many treatments applying this method in a variety of sports. I decided to publish this manual explaining the M-Test method in detail in order to reach a wider audience.

This manual explains in detail the basic concepts needed to apply the theory of meridians and acupuncture points to the analysis of body movements, the study of biomechanics, the distinguishing features of the M-Test, and the relationship between the M-Test and the major muscles of the body. By including many photos and illustrations, we have shown clearly and simply the skills needed for mastering the M-Test method. Furthermore, based on the results of the M-Test, we have explained how the meridians and acupuncture points are selected, and how the M-Test method is applied in cases that are representative of a variety of sports, each with its specific characteristics. In addition to illustrations of the locations of frequently used acupuncture points, we have also included some 'coffee break' stories on interesting topics that make this manual fun to read. In these stories, I asked the practitioners who helped write this manual to share some of their secrets, as well as accounts of their successes and interesting episodes.

My intention is for readers to thumb through the pages of this manual, to read a chapter or a story, whatever captures their interest. Following their curiosity in this way, readers can pick up this method and become familiar with the concept of sports acupuncture using the M-Test before they try it. I look forward to the popularization of this method and to the use of acupuncture in the day-to-day conditioning of athletes and the improvement of their performances, as well as for rehabilitation after injury.

—MUKAINO YOSHITO, M.D.

Professor, Faculty of Sports and Health Science,
* Fukuoka University*
September, 2003

---

1. These acronyms refer to the Commission for University Sports Study (CESU) of the International University Sports Federation (FISU). The original name is in French.

2. An international sports event of university students held every two years at different locations.

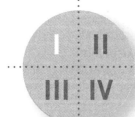

SECTION I

Theoretical Background of Sports Acupuncture

1

CHAPTER 1

· ·

Approach through Meridians and Acupuncture Points

by Mukaino Yoshito, M.D.

A. Analysis and Treatment of Physical Movements

JOINTS ARE THE FOUNDATION of all movements in our body, and they consist of muscles, tendons, ligaments and bones. In modern biomedicine, research and analysis of physical movement has focused mainly on detailed knowledge of individual joints. Movement of any one joint, however, initiates movement in the rest of the body, and each joint is affected by movements of other joints. In an example provided by Keizo Hashimoto, M.D., when we lie on the floor on our back with our feet against the wall and try to push the wall with our big toes, we exert effort in the following order: toes → ankles → knees → hips → spine → shoulders → elbows → wrists → neck. In the end, even our facial muscles become tense. When any restraint is placed on any part of this chain of movement, the coordination of the whole movement is disrupted. Such restraints, or resistance in the system, can cause pain in an area where no injury or restriction existed before. If our analysis of movement is limited to a narrow focus on individual joints, our treatment inevitably ends up being inadequate because we fail to take into account the reciprocal relationship of other joints.

Oriental medicine, with its concept of meridians and acupuncture points, provides a methodology that can be used to analyze the reciprocal relationship of multiple joints in movement. This perspective of interconnection is possible because our bodies are said to have acupuncture points on meridians that are distributed in a vertical

3

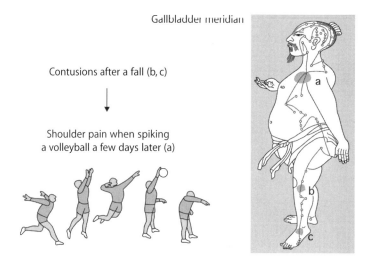

Gallbladder meridian

Contusions after a fall (b, c)

Shoulder pain when spiking
a volleyball a few days later (a)

Symptoms like pain are induced by imbalances in movements of the body as a whole. The mutual influence of multiple joints in movement appears along the longitudinal axis. It is easier to understand the mechanism of the manifestation of symptoms when we apply the concept of meridians.

● **Figure I–1**   Application of meridians to the analysis of movement

pattern from head to toe. Acupuncture points are located bilaterally on the arms and legs, and the meridians are presented as a line or pathway connecting these points. Since these meridians run along the vertical axis of the body, movements can generally be analyzed in terms of connections along these vertical lines.

Let me explain this concept using a case from my clinic. A volleyball player came to me who experienced shoulder pain while spiking the ball (Fig. I–1). I could not find any physical abnormality in the shoulder (a), and I could not explain the mechanism causing the pain. But I learned that, while doing a blocking exercise a few days earlier, this player had taken a fall that caused minor contusions on his knee (b) and the side of his ankle (c). The locations of the contusions corresponded to the acupuncture points GB-40 and GB-34 on the Gallbladder meridian. Even though this player did not experience any discomfort there, these points were extremely tender when pressed. Although acupuncture performed on the shoulder area was ineffective, acupuncture at GB-40 and GB-34 immediately alleviated the shoulder pain. As shown in the figure, it can be seen that the spiking movement that triggered the shoulder pain stretches the muscles on the side of the body (along the Gallbladder meridian in this case). If we think of the contusion in the lower extremity as the origin of the problem that initiated a restriction in the extension of muscles along the Gallbladder meridian, then we can understand

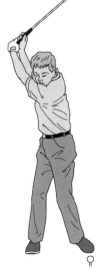

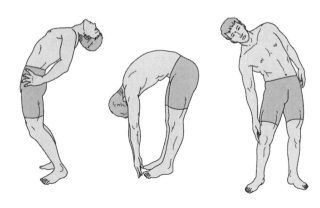

● **Figure I–3** Body balance and meridians during a golf swing

● **Figure I–2** Movement and meridians

how this could be the mechanism that ultimately caused the shoulder pain. When we understand this concept of a chain reaction of restrictions in the extension of muscles along a meridian, then we can apply this mechanism of symptom propagation—the reciprocal relationship of movements across multiple joints—in our practice. Based on this understanding, we can find effective acupuncture points for treating a wide range of musculoskeletal symptoms.

When we take a fresh look at the meridians for the purpose of analyzing the relationship between movements and the body, the meridians can be categorized into three groups: 1) those that can be used to assess the connection between each of the four extremities and the torso; 2) those that that can be used to assess the connection between the upper and lower extremities and the torso; and 3) those that can be used to assess the connection between the central axis of the body and whole body movements. Take for example comparatively simple movements like extension, flexion, and lateral flexion of the torso, as shown in Figure I–2. Each large movement consists of smaller movements of the arms, legs, and torso. Furthermore, each smaller movement influences the other. The three categories of meridians listed above enable us to analyze these reciprocal influences. To analyze movements in a sports activity such as a golf swing (Fig. I–3), one must examine the reciprocal influences among the anterior, posterior, and lateral aspects of the extremities and of the torso in addition to understanding the movement as a whole.

It is also possible to apply the ancient Chinese concept of 'five phases' to understand the interrelationships among the meridians. Application of the principles of the five phases enables us to treat abnormalities caused by disruption of the balance between different meridian groups. In this way, the traditional concept of meridians contains a schematic useful for analyzing movements across multiple joints and for correcting imbalances or restrictions in these movements. (See Section F below for a discussion of the principles of the five phases.)

B. Meridians and their Classifications

Meridians can be classified into three groups based on their location on the body: those on the anterior aspect, those on the posterior aspect, and those on the lateral aspect.[1] Within each of these three meridian groups, there is a meridian located in the center of that aspect of the body (Fig. I–4 to I–6). The meridians that are located in the same aspect are classified together. This classification is shown in Table I–1.

1. Yin and yang meridians

Meridians that are located in areas that the sun shines on when a person gets down on all fours are called yang (sunny) meridians. Meridians that are located in the shaded areas when the person assumes the same posture are called yin (shady) meridians. Among the

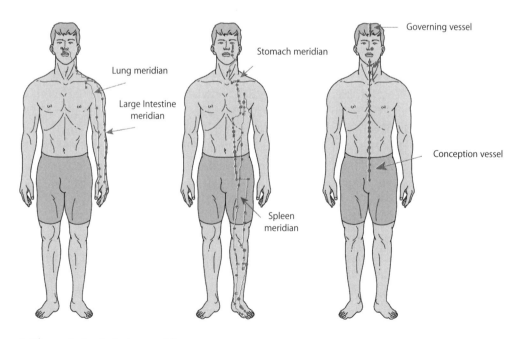

● **Figure I–4**   Anterior meridians

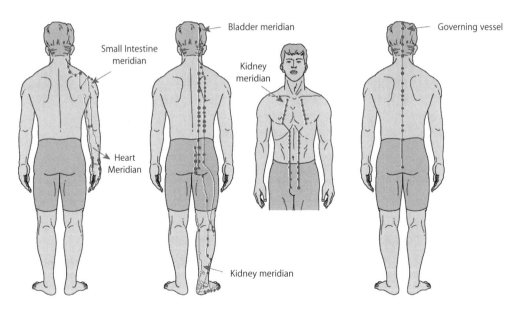

● **Figure I–5** Posterior meridians

twelve regular meridians, six are classified as yin meridians, and the other six are classified as yang meridians.[2]

2. The twelve regular meridians

The meridians that are named after the organs (*zang* and *fu*)[3] of Chinese medicine are called regular meridians. Each of the twelve regular meridians connects to an organ; for example, the Lung meridian connects to the lungs. Each of the six yin organs/meridians connects to one of the yang organs/meridians. The yin-yang organ/meridian pairs are as follows:

YIN (INTERIOR)	YANG (EXTERIOR)
Lungs	Large Intestine
Spleen	Stomach
Heart	Small Intestine
Kidneys	Bladder
Pericardium	Triple Burner
Liver	Gallbladder

3. Exterior-interior meridians

The meridians paired in the yin-yang relationships shown above are also known as exterior-interior meridians. Thus, an 'exterior' yang meridian is paired with an 'interior' yin meridian. There are six such exterior-interior pairs, and each pair is located on opposite aspects of the body. In other words, they are located on the anterior and poste-

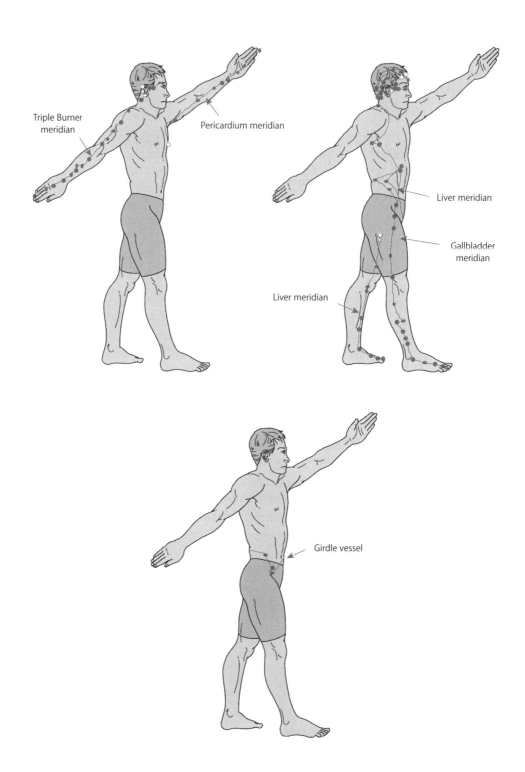

Triple Burner
meridian

Pericardium meridian

Liver meridian

Gallbladder
meridian

Liver meridian

Girdle vessel

• **Figure I–6**   Lateral meridians

rior aspects, or the lateral and medial aspects, of the arms and legs.

The distribution pattern of exterior-interior meridians on the torso is similar. The Kidney meridian on the anterior aspect of the torso is paired with the Bladder meridian on the posterior aspect of the torso. The exterior-interior meridian pair on the lateral and medial aspects of the body is the Liver and Gallbladder meridians. One exterior-interior meridian pair, consisting of the Spleen and Stomach meridians, is located only on the anterior aspect of the torso and the legs.[4]

4. Same-name meridians

There is another category of meridian pairs, which is those that are located on the same aspect of the arms and legs. I call this category of meridians 'same-name meridians'. In this classification, the yin meridians are paired together and the yang meridians are paired together. The yang same-name meridian pairs are classified into three groups according to their location. The Small Intestine meridian, on the posterior aspect of the arms, and the Bladder meridian, on the posterior aspect of the legs, are collectively called the Greater Yang *(Taiyang)* meridians. The Large Intestine meridian, on the anterior aspect of the arms, and the Stomach meridian, on the anterior aspect of the legs, are collectively called the Brilliant Yang (*Yangming*) meridians. The Triple Burner and Gallbladder meridians, in the middle (lateral aspect) of the arms and legs respectively, are collectively called the Lesser Yang *(Shaoyang)* meridians (see Table I–1).

The yin same-name meridian pairs are also classified into three groups according to their location. The Lung meridian on the anterior aspect of the arms and the Spleen meridian on the anterior aspect of the legs are collectively called the Greater Yin *(Taiyin)* meridians. The Heart meridian on the posterior aspect of the arms and the Kidney meridian on the posterior aspect of the legs are collectively called the Lesser Yin *(Shaoyin)* meridians. The Pericardium meridian on the medial aspects of the arms and the Liver meridian on the medial aspects of the legs are collectively called the Absolute Yin *(Jueyin)* meridians (see Table I–1).

5. The Extraordinary meridians

Three of the eight Extraordinary meridians[5] lie on the central axes at the centers of each of the aspects of the torso (anterior, posterior, and lateral). The Conception vessel *(Renmai)* is in the center of the anterior aspect. The Governing vessel *(Dumai)* is in the center of the posterior aspect. The Girdle vessel *(Daimai)* runs horizontally approximately in the center of the lateral aspect (see column on far right of Table I–1). Unlike these three Extraordinary meridians and

Distribution			Same Name	Yin-Interior Distribution	Yang-Exterior Distribution	Same Name	Central Axis
Front			Greater Yin	Lung (Arms) - - - - -Large Intestine (Arms) Spleen (Legs) - - - - - - -Stomach (Legs)		Brilliant Yang	Conception Vessel
Back			Lesser Yin	Heart (Arms) - - - - -Small Intestine (Arms) Kidney (Legs) - - - - - - Bladder (Legs)		Greater Yang	Governing Vessel
Side			Absolute Yin	Pericardium (Arms)- - -Triple Burner (Arms) Liver (Legs) - - - - - - - Gallbladder (Legs)		Lesser Yang	Girdle Vessel

● **Table I–1**   Relationships and locations of meridians

the twelve regular meridians, which are located on a single aspect, the other five Extraordinary meridians are distributed over several aspects of the body. For example, one traverses the anterior and the posterior aspects, while another traverses the posterior and the lateral aspects.

C. Meridians and body movements

1. Yin-yang meridian pairs on the four extremities

The six meridian pairs, of which two pairs each are located on the anterior, posterior, and lateral aspects of the body, are classified into two groups according to their patterns of distribution on the four extremities. In the first group (Group A), the paired meridians run close together and therefore share an identical load simultaneously with a movement. Pairs that belong to this group are the Lung and Large Intestine meridians and the Heart and Small Intestine meridians on the arms, and the Spleen and Stomach meridians and the Kidney and Bladder meridians on the legs. In the second group (Group B), the paired meridians do not run close together but instead run along opposite aspects of the limbs and therefore take on an opposing (agonist-antagonist) load simultaneously with one movement. Pairs that belong to this group are the Triple Burner and Pericardium meridians on the arms and the Gallbladder and Liver meridians on the legs.

As shown in Figure I–7 for Group A, when the wrist is flexed toward the ulna, the Lung meridian (yin), which ends in the tip of the thumb, and the Large Intestine meridian (yang), which starts at the tip of the index finger, share the same extension load. Similarly, when the wrist is flexed toward the radius, the Small Intestine meridian (yang), which starts at the tip of the little finger, and the Heart Meridian (yin), which ends at the tip of the ring finger, share the same extension load.

Furthermore, as shown in Figure I–7 for Group B, when the wrist is flexed, the Triple Burner meridian (yang) is stretched. Conversely, when the wrist is extended, the Pericardium meridian (yin) is stretched. In short, yin-yang meridian pairs consist of two distinct groups. Group A, which consists of the Lung/Large Intestine meridian pair and the Heart/Small Intestine meridian pair, shares an identical or similar load in movement. Group B, which consists of the Triple Burner/Pericardium meridian pair and the Gallbladder/Liver meridian pair, takes on an opposing load. This general rule also applies when evaluating movement of the elbows and shoulders. The same characteristics of Group A and Group B meridian pairs also apply to the lower extremities.

Group A: Exterior-interior meridians located close together. One movement puts a similar load on both meridians.

Group B: Exterior-interior meridians located on opposite sides from each other. One movement puts opposite loads on each meridian.

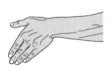
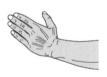
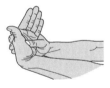
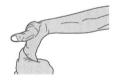

Large Intestine meridian
Lung meridian

Small Intestine meridian
Heart meridian

Triple Burner meridian

Pericardium meridian

● **Figure I–7** Exterior-interior meridian pairs and movement

2. Same-name meridians

Two same-name meridian pairs (one yin pair and one yang pair) are located on each aspect of the body (anterior, posterior, and lateral). So there are three groups, one for each aspect. The yang same-name meridians are called Brilliant Yang *(Yangming)* on the anterior aspect, Greater Yang *(Taiyang)* on the posterior aspect, and Lesser Yang *(Shaoyang)* on the lateral aspects (including the medial aspect).

The yin same-name meridians are called Greater Yin *(Taiyin)* on the anterior aspect, Lesser Yin *(Shaoyin)* on the posterior aspect, and Absolute Yin *(Jueyin)* on the lateral aspects.

Thus the Brilliant Yang meridians are located on the front of the body on the arms, legs, and torso, the Lesser Yang meridians are located on the sides of the body, and the Greater Yang meridians are located on the back of the body. These characteristic locations of same-name yang meridians also hold true on the neck and head, as shown in Figure I–8. Thus the Brilliant Yang meridians (Stomach and Large Intestine) are on the anterior neck, the Lesser Yang meridians (Triple Burner and Gallbladder) are on the lateral neck, and the Greater Yang meridians (Small Intestine and Bladder) are on the posterior neck. Therefore, the Greater Yang meridians are extended when the neck is in flexion, the Brilliant Yang meridians are extended when the neck is in extension, and the Lesser Yang meridians are extended when the neck is flexed laterally. In short, the same-name yang meridian pairs take on an identical load with movement. While the same-name yin meridian pairs are not always located on the same aspects, as with the yang meridian pairs, their relationship is similar to that of the yang meridian pairs.

3. Meridians on the torso

The yin-yang meridian pairs on the torso are located on different aspects than on the lower extremities. Thus the stretch placed on

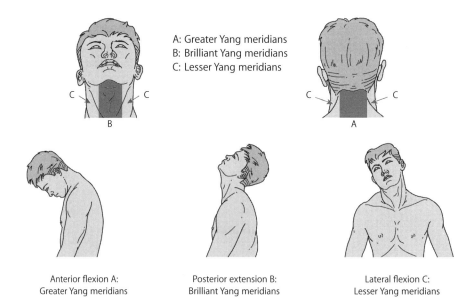

A: Greater Yang meridians
B: Brilliant Yang meridians
C: Lesser Yang meridians

Anterior flexion A:
Greater Yang meridians

Posterior extension B:
Brilliant Yang meridians

Lateral flexion C:
Lesser Yang meridians

● **Figure I–8**   Same-name yang meridians and load of movement

these meridian pairs by extension of the anterior, posterior, and lateral torso is different than the stretch on these meridian pairs in the four extremities. For example, the Kidney and Bladder meridians, which are close to each other on the lower legs, separate on the upper leg and end up on opposite sides of the torso. So on the torso, the Kidney meridian is on the anterior aspect and the Bladder meridian is on the posterior aspect. Conversely, the Liver and Gallbladder meridians are on opposite sides of the lower extremities and run close to each other on the torso. Only the Spleen and Stomach meridians maintain an almost parallel position on both the lower extremities and the torso.

Among the Eight Extraordinary meridians, the Conception vessel, Governing vessel, and Girdle vessel are located in the center of the anterior, posterior, and lateral aspects of the torso. These three meridians are the central axes in each of these aspects. Extension of each aspect of the torso places a load on the axial Extraordinary meridian. Since ancient times the axial meridians, especially the Conception and Governing vessels, have been defined as meridians that regulate the other meridians. The Girdle vessel, which encircles the midsection of the torso like a belt, can be viewed as serving the role of an axial meridian for the lateral aspects of the body.

D. Meridians, Acupuncture Points, and Physical Movement

1. Characteristics of acupuncture points and their locations

Most acupuncture points are located in areas of the body where muscles and tendons attach to the bones, between tendons, at joints, on the bellies of muscles, or on areas surrounding blood vessels. It is surmised that stimulating acupuncture points improves circulation and facilitates movement in the surrounding muscles, tendons, and joints. Concurrently, the influence of this stimulation is transmitted to the whole body via the meridian on which the acupuncture point is located.

Acupuncture points are classified into several groups, including the essential points on the four extremities representing each meridian. Among the essential points are the Associated *(shu)* points located on the back, and the Alarm *(mu)* points located on the chest and abdomen. Each of these points relates closely to the movement of the meridians as well as to the body as a whole (see Fig. I–9).

2. Roles of meridians and acupuncture points during meridian extension

a. Yin-yang meridian pairs

The relationship between the extension (stretching) of a meridian and

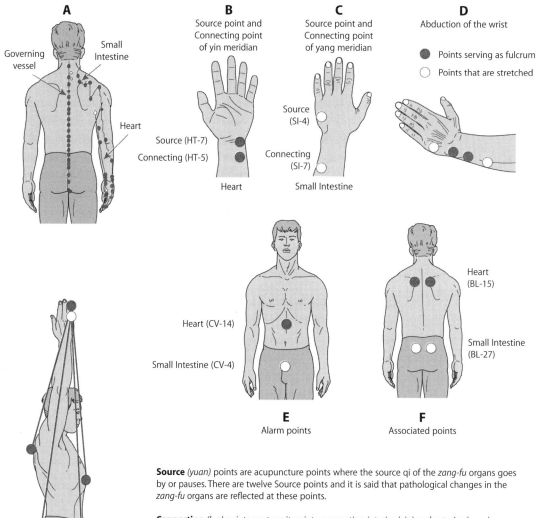

A

Governing vessel

Small Intestine

Heart

B
Source point and Connecting point of yin meridian

Source (HT-7)

Connecting (HT-5)

Heart

C
Source point and Connecting point of yang meridian

Source (SI-4)

Connecting (SI-7)

Small Intestine

D
Abduction of the wrist

● Points serving as fulcrum

○ Points that are stretched

Heart (CV-14)

Small Intestine (CV-4)

Heart (BL-15)

Small Intestine (BL-27)

E
Alarm points

F
Associated points

G
Relationship between shoulder flexion and Associated and Alarm points

Source *(yuan)* points are acupuncture points where the source qi of the *zang-fu* organs goes by or pauses. There are twelve Source points and it is said that pathological changes in the *zang-fu* organs are reflected at these points.

Connecting *(luo)* points are transit points connecting interior (yin) and exterior (yang) meridians. Therefore, when a Connecting point is stimulated, both the interior and exterior meridian are affected.

Associated *(shu)* points are located on the back and are named after the six *zang* and six *fu* organs. There are twelve such points since each *zang-fu* organ is related to a meridian. It is said that the qi of the *zang-fu* organs courses through the Associated points, and they can be used to adjust insufficiency of qi in the *zang-fu* organs. These points become reactive when there is pathology in their associated *zang-fu* organ, so they are important points for diagnosing and treating the *zang-fu* organs.

Alarm *(mu)* points, located on the chest and abdominal area, are said to be where the qi of the *zang-fu* organs collects. There are twelve Alarm points. They are as important as Associated points for diagnosing and treating pathological changes in the *zang-fu* organs. The Alarm points and Associated points of the same organ are located at almost the same level on the anterior and posterior aspects of the body. The Alarm points on the front and Associated points on the back presumably function as the counterpoints on the torso in the extension of related meridians.

● **Figure I–9**   Source, Connecting, Associated, and Alarm points: Relationship of the Heart-Small Intestine meridians and Governing vessel

the Source *(yuan)* point, the Connecting *(luo)* point, the Associated *(shu)* point, and the Alarm *(mu)* point of a yin-yang meridian pair is shown in Figure I–9, using the Heart and Small Intestine meridians as an example. In this figure, (A) shows the paths of the Heart and Small Intestine meridians, which run close together on the posterior aspect of the arms. Because of their proximity, both of these meridians are affected in the same way by a particular movement. HT-7, the Source point of the yin Heart meridian, is located near the wrist joint, as shown in (B). SI-4, the Source point of the yang Small Intestine meridian, is more distal than HT-7, as shown in (C). When the wrist joint is flexed radially, as shown in (D), the yin-yang meridian pair of the Heart and Small Intestine is stretched. HT-7 becomes a fulcrum in this movement and stretches the area where SI-4 is located. This means, in the case of radial flexion of the wrist, that the Source point of the yin meridian becomes the fulcrum and the Source point of the yang meridian is stretched. The location of Connecting points follows almost the same principle, but SI-7, the Connecting point of the Small Intestine meridian, is located more proximally than HT-5, the Connecting point of the Heart meridian (D). Because of this relationship, stimulation of the Source and Connecting points of the yin-yang meridian pairs traversing the wrist improves the movement of the wrist as well as a broader area above and below.

The Associated *(shu)* and Alarm *(mu)* points of the Heart and Small Intestine meridians are located on the back and front of the torso; see (E) and (F) in Figure I–9. The Associated and Alarm points are not usually located on their affiliated meridians, yet each represents a specific meridian. Let us examine the relationship between the Heart and Small Intestine meridians and their Associated and Alarm points on the torso during flexion of the shoulder, as shown in (G). The area of the Heart and Small Intestine meridians on the arm are stretched, and simultaneously, the influence of this movement extends down to the torso. The points on the posterior torso that are connected to this arm movement are the Associated points of the Heart (BL-15) and Small Intestine (BL-27) meridians. I call these points that are connected to and support the movements in other parts of the body 'corresponding points.' The Alarm points of the Heart (CV-14) and Small Intestine (CV-4) meridians, located on the abdomen, serve as the corresponding points on the anterior torso in the same manner as the Associated points do on the back.

In addition to the Associated and Alarm points, there is the Governing vessel of the Extraordinary meridians located on the posterior torso. This meridian serves as the central axis for movements that stretch the Heart and Small Intestine meridians, which are on the posterior aspect. These relationships between meridians, corresponding points, and movement are seen in the other yin-yang meridian pairs on the arms and legs as well.

b. Same-name meridians

The same-name meridian pairs have a relationship that is similar to that of the yin-yang meridian pairs described above. Figure I–10 shows an example of stretching the Brilliant Yang meridians (Large Intestine and Stomach) and the Greater Yin meridians (Lung and Spleen). The extension of the torso shown in this figure stretches the anterior aspect of the torso as well as the arms and the legs. The Brilliant Yang and Greater Yin meridian pairs (Large Intestine/Stomach and Lung/Spleen), which are located on the anterior aspects of the arms and legs, also take on the stress of this extension. The corresponding points on the posterior aspect of the torso in relation to this movement would be the Associated points of the Large Intestine (BL-25), Stomach (BL-21), Lungs (BL-13), and Spleen (BL-20). Similarly, the Alarm points of the Spleen (LV-13), Stomach (CV-12), Lungs (LU-1), and Large Intestine (ST-25) are located on the anterior aspect of

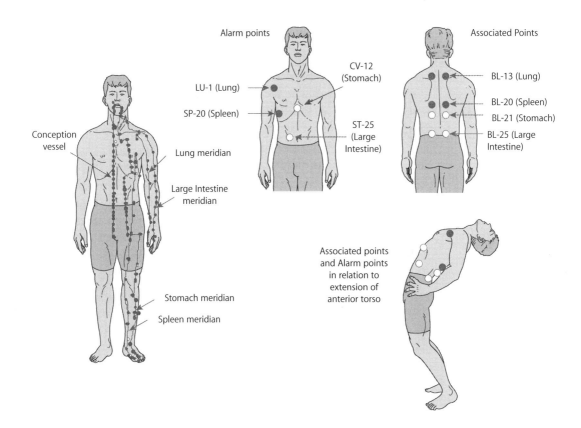

● **Figure I–10**   Stretch of same-name meridians in relation to the Associated and Alarm points

the torso, and serve their role as corresponding points on the anterior aspect. In addition to the Alarm points, the Conception vessel (one of the Extraordinary meridians) is located on the anterior torso and serves as the central axis when the Brilliant Yang meridians (Stomach and Large Intestine) and Greater Yin meridians (Lung and Spleen) are extended. These same relationships between corresponding points on the anterior and posterior aspects and the axial meridian can be observed on the same-name meridian pairs located on the lateral and posterior aspects of the body.

E. Basic Scheme of Meridians and Acupuncture Points (Fig. I–11)

Understanding the system of yin-yang meridian pairs enables us to analyze the linkage of movements in the torso to the arms or the legs. Understanding the same-name meridian pairs enables us to analyze the linkage of movements in the torso to that in the arms and the legs. Understanding the axial Extraordinary meridians (the Conception, Governing, and Girdle vessels) allows us to analyze the relationships between yin-yang meridian pairs or same-name meridian pairs to the central axes on the torso. The acupuncture points located on these related meridians serve to regulate these reciprocal relationships. The principles of the five phases provide another way of analyzing these reciprocal relationships.

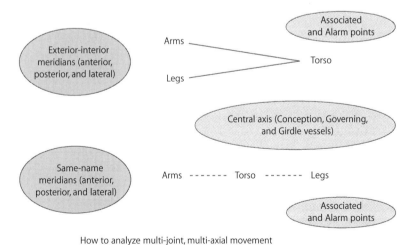

How to analyze multi-joint, multi-axial movement

● **Figure I–11**   Basic organization of meridians and acupuncture points

F. Movement and the five phases

The principles of the five phases is an ancient Chinese ideology that classifies all phenomena in the natural world as products of the interaction of five types (or phases) of matter. The five phases are wood, fire, earth, metal, and water. This principle is also applied to the characteristics and functions of the organs in the human body; thus each organ is classified as wood, fire, earth, metal, or water. This system is used to explain the mutually assisting and mutually constraining relationships between the *zang-fu* organs. The mutually assisting relationship is called the 'generating cycle,' and the mutually constraining relationship is called the 'controlling cycle' (Fig. I–12).

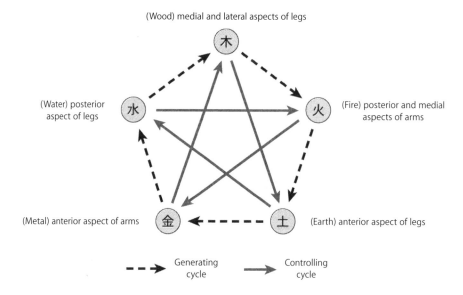

● **Figure I–12**   Relationships between generating and controlling cycles of the five phases and the distribution of meridians

Movements of the human body can also be classified according to the five-phase principles. Wood is associated with the Liver and Gallbladder meridians, which are located in the medial and lateral aspects of the lower extremities. Fire is associated with the Heart, Small Intestine, Pericardium, and Triple Burner meridians. These meridians are respectively located in the posterior aspects of the upper extremities (Heart, Small Intestine) and the medial (Pericardium) and lateral (Triple Burner) aspects of the upper extremities. Earth is associated with the Spleen and Stomach meridians, which are located on the anterior aspects of the lower extremities. Metal is associated with the Lung and Large Intestine meridians, which are located on the anterior aspects of the upper extremities. Finally, water is associated with the Kidney and Bladder meridians, which are located on the posterior aspects of the lower extremities.

Observing these relationships in the movement shown in Figure I–13, we can see that this backbending movement tends to extend or stretch the anterior aspects of the arms and legs, while simultaneously causing contraction in the posterior aspects of the arms and legs. The stretched anterior aspect of the arm is the domain of the Lung and Large Intestine meridians, which are associated with the metal phase. The stretched aspect of the legs is the domain of the Spleen and Stomach meridians, which are associated with the earth phase. The contracted posterior aspect of the arms is the domain of the Heart and Small Intestine meridians, which are associated with the fire phase. The contracted posterior aspect of the legs is the domain of the Kidney and Bladder meridians, which are associated with the water phase. Thus this backbend involves at least four phases, and each of these phases is in generating and controlling relationships.

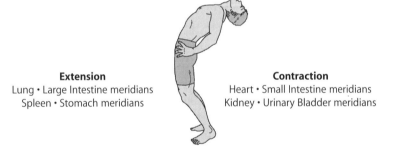

Extension
Lung • Large Intestine meridians
Spleen • Stomach meridians

Contraction
Heart • Small Intestine meridians
Kidney • Urinary Bladder meridians

● **Figure I–13**   Relationship of meridians to movement

In this way, we can use the principles of the five phases to analyze the dynamic movements in sports activities. The yin-yang meridian pairs have six areas of distribution in each arm and leg. One of the interesting characteristics of the meridian distribution on the body is that two meridians each are located on the little finger and the big toe. The little finger plays the most important role in smooth and precise movements of the upper half of the body in actions such as swinging a bat in baseball, a racquet in tennis, and a bamboo sword in kendo fencing. Similarly, the big toe plays an important role when the lower half of the body moves in response to the movements of the upper half. To accomplish any smooth movement, a harmonious linkage between the upper and lower halves of the body is required. The two meridians located on the little finger are the Heart and Small Intestine meridians, and the meridians on the big toe are the Spleen and Liver meridians. According to five-phase principles, the Heart and the Small Intestine are both associated with fire, the Spleen with earth, and the Liver with wood, respectively. The relationships between wood and fire, and fire and earth, are 'generating,' while that between wood and earth is 'controlling' (Fig. I–12).

We can incorporate these relationships into our analysis of the reciprocal relationships between the movements of the arms and legs. Figure I–14 shows the sequential movement of a golf swing. When we observe the extended aspects of the arms and legs in (A), (B), (C), and (D), we see that the lateral (Triple Burner), medial (Pericardium), and posterior (Heart/Small Intestine) aspects are extended or stretched. In other words, the fire aspects of both the right and left upper arms are stretched. On the other hand, the aspects extended or stretched on the legs are different on the right and left sides. In (A) the left leg is stretched on the medial aspect (wood: Liver meridian), while the right leg is stretched on the lateral aspect (wood: Gallbladder meridian). In (C) the left leg is stretched on the lateral aspect (wood: Gallbladder meridian), and the right lower extremity is stretched mainly on the anterior aspect (earth: Spleen and Stomach). In (B), as in (C), the left leg is stretched on the lateral aspect, and the right leg starts to get stretched on the anterior aspect. Also in (D), even though the movement differs from (C), the same aspects are stretched.

In this manner, we can apply five-phase theory to help us understand balance and imbalance in the movements of the arms and legs as we observe sequential movements in sports activities. For example,

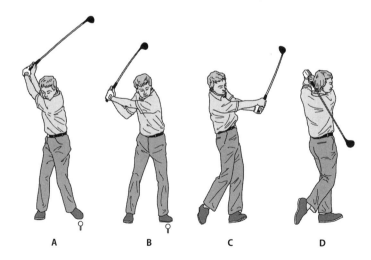

● **Figure I–14**   Sequential movements during a golf swing

if a golfer experiences a problem such as pain or discomfort in (A), we can regard it as an abnormality in the fire aspect (the lateral/medial and posterior aspects of the arms) as well as the wood aspect (the medial and lateral aspects of the legs). When, as in (C), the right leg and the left leg perform different roles, the analysis of the movement must take into account the reciprocal relationship between the arms and legs on each side. Thus in (C), on the right side it is a relationship of fire (lateral and posterior aspects of the arm) and earth (anterior aspect of the leg), and on the left side it is a relationship of fire and wood (lateral aspect of the leg). By performing the Meridian Test (see Part II), one can identify the restrictions in various aspects and understand the problem in movement in terms of the five-phase relationships.

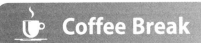

Coffee Break

A Herniated Disk Due to Acupuncture Treatment

Moriyama Tomomasa, Professor of the Tsukuba College of Technology

Back when I was still a novice acupuncturist, a 22-year-old woman came to me for acupuncture for low back pain. Since she didn't have any neurological signs associated with her back pain, I decided that her problem was obviously myofascial strain. I found tension in the lower sacrospinous muscles from the third lumbar vertebra to the area of the second sacral vertebra. In my clinical experience, excessive tension in skeletal muscles must be reduced in order to resolve back pain—this patient's chief complaint. After explaining my assessment to the patient, without hesitation I proceeded to apply low frequency electro-acupuncture to the tense areas. After about 15 minutes of electro-acupuncture, her symptoms improved by almost 70 percent. When she arrived at my clinic, her body stooped forward as she walked, but when she left, she walked normally, clearly having regained her natural posture and movements.

About ten minutes after she left, my clinic phone rang. It was my patient calling, asking for help because she had suffered a sudden attack of low back pain. It hit her as she walked up two or three steps at the train station, and she could not move. I raced over to the station, and drove her to the nearest orthopedic specialist. The doctor diagnosed her with a herniated disk. This case taught me a lesson: Strong local stimulation must be applied with utmost caution for acute patients with weak muscles. •

References

1. Hashimoto Keizo and Kawakami Yoshiaki, *SOTAI: Balance and Health Through Natural Movement*, Japan Publications, 1983.
2. Mukaino Yoshito, Gerald Kolblinger, and Chen Yong, *Keiraku Tesuto* (Meridian Test), Ishiyaku Shuppan, 1999.
3. Mukaino Yoshito, *Keiraku Tesuto ni Yoru Shindan to Hari Chiryo* (Diagnosis and Acupunture Treatment Using the Meridian Test), Ishiyaku Shuppan, 2002.

Notes

1. The anatomical position in Oriental medicine is different from that of Western medicine. It is defined as standing at attention with the arms hanging at the sides of the body, the palms facing the body and the thumbs forward. Anterior refers to the areas seen from the front of the standing person, and posterior refers to the areas seen from the back. Lateral refers to the areas seen from the side. The sides of the arms and legs that can't be seen because they are facing the body are the medial aspects.

2. Yin and yang: The complementary opposites of yin and yang are used in Chinese medicine to describe all aspects of anatomy and physiology. There is no absolute yin independent of yang; yin always contains some yang and vice versa. When yin reaches its extremity, it changes into yang. Yin pertains to shade, night, cold, water, and the feminine quality. Yang pertains to daytime, heat, fire, and the masculine quality.

3. *Zang* and *fu*: The *zang* are yin organs that are located in the 'interior' of the body. There are six *zang*: Lungs, Spleen, Heart, Kidneys, Pericardium, and Liver. The *fu* are yang organs that are located in the 'exterior' or more superficial level of the body. There are six *fu* organs: Large Intestine, Stomach, Small Intestine, Bladder, Triple Burner, and Gallbladder. The Triple Burner is an organ with no defined form. It is described as follows in Chapter 31 of the *Classic of Difficulties* (*Nan Jing*, c. 1st or 2nd century A.D.): "The Triple Burner is the passage of water and grain, where qi [vital energy] begins and ends." The Triple Burner is thus a *fu* organ involved in all of the digestive functions, including water metabolism. The structure and functions of the organs in Chinese medicine were derived from speculation, so in many cases they do not correspond with the organs of the same name in Western medicine. It is therefore best to consider the *zang* and *fu* as being fundamentally different from their Western counterparts, and for this reason, we will capitalize them in this book.

4. The Stomach meridian: Even though the Stomach meridian is yang (sunny), it is located on the anterior or yin (shady) aspect of the torso. The location of the yang Stomach meridian on the anterior aspect is an exception to the rule. There is no good explanation for this. In Chinese medical theory, the Stomach is an essential organ that life itself depends on, and it is considered inseparable from the Spleen.

5. Eight Extraordinary meridians: Conception vessel, Governing vessel, Girdle vessel, Penetrating vessel, Yang Linking vessel, Yin Linking vessel, Yang Heel vessel, and Yin Heel vessel. The Extraordinary meridians were viewed as connecting and regulating pathways for the regular meridians. According to the *Yellow Emperor's Inner Classic*, "Extraordinary meridians are like ditches that hold water overflowing from the rivers." Thus, they are usually called 'vessels' instead of meridians.

· ·

CHAPTER 2

A Biomechanical Approach

by Moriyama Tomomasa

A. The Use of Acupuncture to Improve Body Movement

1) USING ACUPUNCTURE TO TREAT A WORLD-RANKED TENNIS PLAYER

IN 1992 I WENT TO THE 25th Olympic Games in Barcelona as one of the trainers for the Japanese tennis team. I looked after the physical conditioning of the players, and I used acupuncture as one of the methods to improve their conditioning. Figure I–15 is a photo of an acupuncture treatment. Tennis player M arrived at the Athletes' Village from Japan with a sprain of the metatarsophalangeal joint of the left big toe. After he practiced, I applied ice to the affected area, and then needled the peroneus longus muscle on the lateral aspect of the leg to relieve the excess tension in the muscle and to prevent the effect of the sprain from spreading to the shoulders. Tennis player M was ranked 46th in the world, and was especially skillful at the offensive game of serve-and-volley; he was able to consistently serve the ball at speeds exceeding 180 km/h (113 mph).

I will explain the theoretical basis of treatment, how to analyze body movements specific to a sports activity, the method of applying this approach to acupuncture treatments, and the rationale for the treatment. Acupuncture treatments are by no means performed only empirically. The results from accumulated clinical experience are being studied scientifically in Japan today. This is the time for acupuncture in the field of sports to take a bold leap from merely treating injuries to the prevention of injuries, and beyond that, to improving the conditioning and performance of athletes.

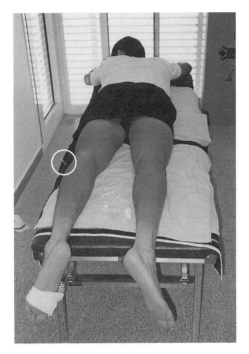

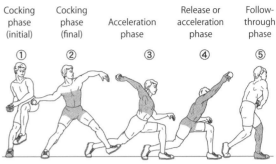

Cocking phase (initial)	Cocking phase (final)	Acceleration phase	Release or acceleration phase	Follow-through phase
①	②	③	④	⑤

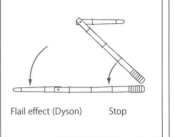

Flail effect (Dyson)   Stop

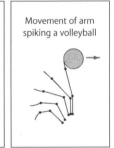

Movement of arm spiking a volleyball

● **Figure I–15**
Acupuncture treatment for conditioning

● **Figure I–16** Pitching phases and the structure of joint movements (flail effect)

2) Using biomechanics to analyze body movements

a. The basic concept: How to understand joint movement and movement in the entire body (are they dynamically balanced?)

(1) Analyzing single joint movements

When we carefully observe a large movement involving the entire body, we see the joints become fixed one after another in order to enable the next joint to move. This phenomenon is called kinetic setting. Many joints are involved in the throwing of a baseball. Even if we limit our observation to the upper half of the body, the throwing movement starts from the neck and trunk, and goes on to the shoulder, elbow, and wrist. The joints become sequentially fixed, starting with the trunk (the core). An efficient and beautiful form is created only after this sequential kinetic setting. A British exercise physiologist, G. Dyson, called this the "flail-like action" (Fig. I–16).

(2) Analyzing the linkage of multiple joint movements

In a similar manner, when standing upright, energy from the lower half of the body is transmitted to the upper body. The force of movement transmits through the soles and the joints of the feet to the lower legs and the knee joints, the thighs and the hip joints, and finally up to the lumbar area (the core). Many researchers have measured the speed of movement in the joints of the trunk and joints in the four extremities to analyze the energy efficiency of movements according to variations in the transmission sequence. It has been concluded that it is most energy efficient to use many joints and to move the arm as if it were a whip (Fig. I–17).

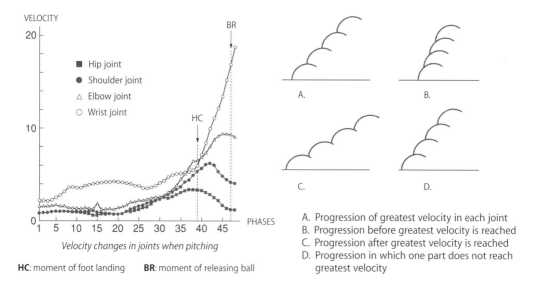

VELOCITY

■ Hip joint
● Shoulder joint
△ Elbow joint
○ Wrist joint

HC

BR

PHASES

Velocity changes in joints when pitching

HC: moment of foot landing   **BR**: moment of releasing ball

A. Progression of greatest velocity in each joint
B. Progression before greatest velocity is reached
C. Progression after greatest velocity is reached
D. Progression in which one part does not reach greatest velocity

● **Figure I–17**   Graph of energy conduction in movement of joints (velocity change) and angular velocity of body segments

(Laurence Morehouse & John Cooper, *Kinesiology*, Kimpton, 1950)

This hypothesis gives us an important clue to the clinical practice of acupuncture. In cases of sports injuries caused by overuse of the muscles, we tend to pay attention to the joints that undergo strenuous movement. Actually, we must also pay attention to the joints that stabilize the area of strenuous movement. These constitute the axis of the movement. This implies that injuries can occur because the strength to stabilize the most active joint is not sufficient. The strength to stabilize or fix a joint must increase in proportion to the power of the forceful movement. A balance between the strength to stabilize and the power to move prevents injury. The key to conditioning and improving performance lies in understanding the characteristics of movements in various sports, and the ability to balance stabilizing strength with powerful movements in a particular situation. I will give an example of applying biomechanics in conditioning for athletes using acupuncture, and explain how acupuncture treatment can lead to improvement in the athlete's performance.

b. An example of diagnosis and treatment: The linkage between the pelvic girdle, the lumbar region, the neck and shoulder, and the arms

(1) How the collapse of the plantar arch and ankle deformity influences the lower limb and lumbar region

As the most distal parts of our lower limbs, the feet contact the ground during locomotion, and the calves and the ankle joints assist in supporting the weight of the body. Explaining this function in terms of the concept of the "flail-like action" mentioned above, the knee joints are the parts that fixate to stabilize the limb and allow maximum movement in distal joints.

> ✔ CHECK POINTS ON THE FOOT
> a) Collapse of the plantar arch
> b) Talipes valgus: pronation of ankle (leg-heel alignment)
> c) Hallux valgus: lateral displacement of big toe

The problem that is common to all of these conditions is the collapse of the plantar arch (the sinking of the navicular bone). In Japanese, the plantar arch is called *tsuchi fumazu*, which literally means 'not stepping on earth'. This clearly portrays the plantar arch, which curves like a bow and does not contact the ground when we walk with bare feet. Why does this arch exist and what is its function?

The flatfoot is one that does not have much of an arch. Traditionally, the flatfoot has been synonymous with quickly becoming fatigued from walking. In fact, until recently, we rarely saw flatfeet in the top athletes, except in special cases with hereditary factors. Recently, however, when we performed medical check-ups on the junior athletes in Japan, we noticed some players with flatfeet or hallux valgus (lateral displacement of the big toe). It is said that the formation of the plantar arch is complete by the age of six or seven. The primary function of this arch is to act as a shock absorber. Because of this arch, the bones of the foot are not crushed even when the feet must counteract gravity at increasing speeds to support the weight of the body. This means that the plantar arch is designed to adjust its shape from high to low according to the intensity of physical activity. Over time, however, as an athlete constantly walks, runs, and jumps, the height of the plantar arch is gradually reduced. This, in other words, is plantar fatigue. When an athlete continues to play a sport with a lowered arch, it causes plantar fasciitis, which can develop into other injuries. The skeletal muscles that lift this bony arch are the tibialis posterior and peroneus longus. These muscles have their insertions in the navicular and medial cuneiform bones. A decline in the elevation (upward traction) of the navicular bone can cause many injuries (Fig. I–18).

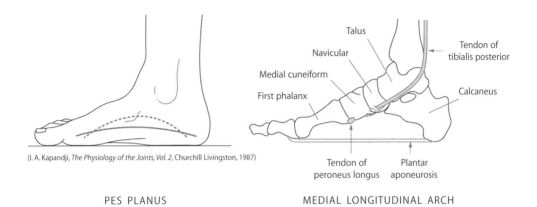

(I. A. Kapandji, *The Physiology of the Joints, Vol. 2*, Churchill Livingston, 1987)

PES PLANUS   MEDIAL LONGITUDINAL ARCH

● **Figure I-18**   Flatfoot and medial plantar arch

The condition of hallux valgus causes pronation and medial displacement of the ankle joint. The medial aspect of the foot is extended when the great toe is displaced laterally, and this tends to cause pronation of the ankle joint. The plantar arch decreases as the ankle becomes pronated. This medial displacement of the ankle also causes lateral rotation of the lower leg and excess tension in quadriceps femoris, which increases the quadriceps angle (Q-angle), as shown in Figure I–19. Excess tension in the quadriceps femoris causes abnormalities in the 'lumbopelvic rhythm' (i.e., anterior rotation of the pelvis) and creates excess lumbar lordosis, which can lead to lumbago. Also, an increase in the quadriceps angle can lead to knee injuries.

  ✔ CHECK POINTS AROUND THE KNEES
  a) Quadriceps angle (Q-angle)
  b) Excessive tension in quadriceps and tensor fasciae latae
  c) Excessive tension in piriformis and saritorius
  d) Lateral rotation of the lower leg

(2) Abnormalities in 'lumbopelvic rhythm' are caused by imbalances in the lumbar and leg muscles.

The term 'lumbopelvic rhythm' refers to the normal lordosis of the lumbar vertebrae, which depends on the rotation of the pelvic girdle. It indicates the movement and the linkage between the lumbar vertebrae and the pelvic girdle. Physiologically, the pelvis is in anterior

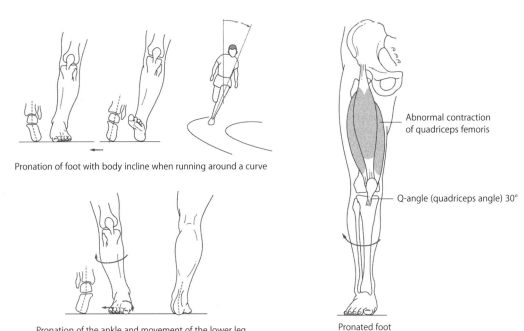

Pronation of foot with body incline when running around a curve

Pronation of the ankle and movement of the lower leg

(Steven Subotnick, *Podiatric Sports Medicine*, 2nd ed., Futura Publishing, 1979)

Abnormal contraction of quadriceps femoris

Q-angle (quadriceps angle) 30°

Pronated foot

● **Figure I–19**   Lateral rotation of lower leg with pronation of foot and influence on thigh

rotation (anteversion). The angle between the pelvis and the fifth lumbar vertebra just above the sacrum is called the lumbosacral angle. An increase in the lumbosacral angle increases the lordosis in the lumbar vertebrae, which also reduces the posterior spaces of the intervertebral disks. This can cause low back pain.

The downward rotation of the anterior aspect of the pelvis, or the anterior superior iliac spine, is called the anterior rotation (anteversion) of the pelvis. This downward rotation of the pelvis increases the lumbosacral angle. Therefore, an abnormality in the 'lumbopelvic rhythm' means nothing other than excessive anterior rotation of the pelvis. The primary factors that cause the anterior rotation of the pelvis are listed below; see also Figure I–20.

↙ CHECK POINTS FOR THE LUMBAR REGION
a) Excessive tension in erector spinae (and sacrospinalis)
b) Insufficient muscle tone in rectus abdominis
c) Insufficient muscle tone in gluteus maximus
d) Excessive tension in tensor fasciae latae and the rectus femoris
e) Loss of elasticity in iliopsoas

These issues can be addressed directly with acupuncture. Reducing

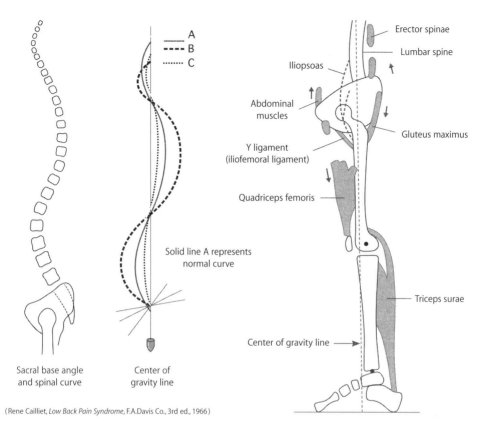

A
B
C

Erector spinae

Lumbar spine

Iliopsoas

Abdominal
muscles

Gluteus maximus

Y ligament
(iliofemoral ligament)

Quadriceps femoris

Solid line A represents
normal curve

Triceps surae

Center of gravity line

Sacral base angle
and spinal curve

Center of
gravity line

(Rene Cailliet, *Low Back Pain Syndrome*, F.A.Davis Co., 3rd ed., 1966)

● **Figure I–20**   Changes in spinal curve and muscle related to lumbopelvic rhythm

tension in excessively tense muscle serves as treatment. It should be noted here that the use of acupuncture in athletes should not be limited to treatment in the narrow sense, but should also serve as a vehicle for conditioning. At the very least, it must include some advice on muscle strength training. Furthermore, when you serve as a trainer for an athlete, you must have a deep insight into optimal performance, which is a result of balance in the whole body. When we actually treat athletes, we must make them understand the aims of our treatment in relation to their particular circumstances. Acupuncture treatment in athletes is almost always contraindicated just before a game. In giving treatments we have to adapt to the circumstances, and possess the knowledge and ability to choose the best approach and techniques, and vary the amount of stimulation according to the receptivity of the athlete to acupuncture.

The above check points a) to e) can occur simultaneously, but depending on an athlete's situation, only a few may be identified. Therefore, in order to understand which muscles need a reduction in tension and which muscles need strengthening, we must observe the balance of muscle tone in the whole body and the muscles' functionality in movement.

(3) Abnormalities in the 'scapulohumeral rhythm' and pain in the neck-shoulder region

The abnormalities in 'lumbopelvic rhythm' mentioned above create tension in the latissimus dorsi, which originates in the lumbar region. Tension in the latissimus dorsi simultaneously causes tension in the teres major, and limits the movement of the scapula during movements of the shoulder joint. In sports injuries involving shoulder problems, there is often a problem with abduction, extension, medial rotation, or lateral rotation. In cases like this, it is necessary to determine if there is any abnormality in the interconnected movements of the scapula and the humerus. In other words, the 'scapulohumeral rhythm' must be examined. Examining the degree of movement in the scapula in relation to movements of the humerus allows us to determine whether there is narrowing in the glenohumeral joint space. Signs of impingement syndrome will appear if the extent of this narrowing increases.

The concept of a 'scapulohumeral rhythm' is predicated on the floating or free movement of the scapula over the ribcage. When there is tension of the latissimus dorsi or the teres major as discussed above, this causes a downward fixation of the scapula, and adduction and extension of the shoulder joint is compromised (Fig. I–21). When the shoulder joint must be moved while the movement of the scapula is restricted by an external cause such as this, the outer muscles represented by the deltoid are forced to work harder. This causes an

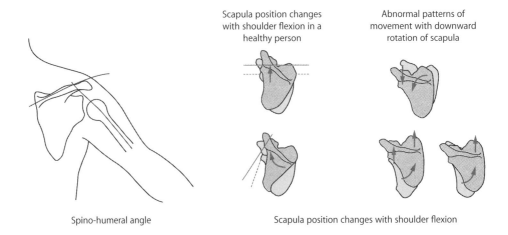

Scapula position changes with shoulder flexion in a healthy person

Abnormal patterns of movement with downward rotation of scapula

Spino-humeral angle

Scapula position changes with shoulder flexion

● **Figure I–21**   Normal and abnormal patterns in scapulohumeral rhythm (from Tsutsui et. al.)

imbalance with the inner muscles, represented by the rotator muscles, which compose the rotator cuff. This, in turn, produces abnormalities in the 'scapulohumeral rhythm.'

> ✔ CHECK POINTS IN THE NECK-SHOULDER SECTION
> a) Excessive tension in the latissimus dorsi and the teres major
> b) Abnormality of the 'scapulohumeral rhythm'
> c) Muscle tone in the rotator muscles

The rotator cuff holds the head of the humerus in place while the shoulder joint moves. In other words, it exerts a downward force on the humerus and holds it in the inferior position, which keeps the glenohumoral joint space open. When the transmission of the kinetic energy from the pelvic girdle up toward the shoulder joint is insufficient, the excessive effort of the shoulder girdle in isolation causes fatigue in the muscles around the shoulder. In shoulder movements, the head of the humerus tends to press up against the acromion, especially when the functionality of the rotator muscles is diminished. This is true when there is weakness in the prime movers for lateral rotation of the shoulder joint (infraspinatus and teres minor) or the prime mover for medial rotation (subscapularis). This leads to pain and restriction in range of motion in the shoulder.

The strategy for acupuncture treatment of shoulder injuries can be determined based on the perspective of biomechanics, as detailed above. When there is shoulder pain due to narrowing of the glenohumoral joint space, steps must be taken to reduce the tension in the outer muscles along with treatment for the functional recuperation of the rotator cuff. Furthermore, we must find where the transmission of energy from the pelvic girdle to the shoulder girdle is being restricted and treat this area. In order to examine and treat athletes in this way, we must always observe the entire body and overall condition. We need to understand all the factors in the athlete's performance, and strive to create a better environment for the athlete, including the training staff.

Everything discussed above is shown in Table I–2. Literally, just having hallux valgus (lateral displacement of big toe) can cause shoulder pain. Hidden under the shoulder pain, there is often a collapsed plantar arch. The functional deterioration in the foot and leg can lead to shoulder pain. Do not examine shoulder pain without looking into the functionality of the feet and legs. This is the same as saying, "Do not look at the illness without paying attention to the patient." This is the essence of Oriental medicine.

(4) Examination from the perspective of Oriental medicine

Considering our clinical approach based on the above discussion, it is clear that we must include the conditioning of the lower limbs

Mechanism of Shoulder and Low Back Pain	Conditioning / Acupuncture Treatment
1. Inverted leg (leg-heel alignment) 2. *Hallux valgus* 3. *Metatarsus latus*	Observation of structure and characteristic movements
↓	↓
Sinking of plantar arch (reversible flat feet) Plantar fascitis	Use of arch supports Massage plantar arch* Acupuncture to relieve fatigue in foot
↓	↓
Excessive tension in tibialis posterior and peroneus longus (shin splints, tibial periosteitis)	Acupuncture to relieve fatigue of tibialis posterior Acupuncture to relieve fatigue of peroneus longus
↓	↓
Stress on medial and lateral knee (fissure in medial femur, pain in medial collateral ligament)	Acupuncture to alleviate pain in the knee and improve circulation around the knee
↓	↓
Tension in lateral thigh (rectus femoris and iliotibial band) Increase in Q-angle, and malalignment of leg bones	Acupuncture on rectus femoris and tensor fasciae latae Strength training for biceps femoris
↓	
Abnormality in "lumbopelvic rhythm" Anterior rotation of pelvis	Acupuncture on iliopsoas and sacro-spinous muscles Strength training for rectus abdominus and gluteus
↓	↓
Increase in lumbar lordosis (excessive tension in iliopsoas, erector spinae, and latissimus dorsi)	Exercises to reduce lumbar lordosis and encourage posterior rotation of pelvis
↓	↓
Onset of lumbago. Downward traction of scapula with shoulder movement	Exercises to balance pelvic girdle Acupuncture on latissimus dorsi
↓	↓
Abnormity in 'scapulohumeral rhythm' (functional deterioration of rotator muscles)	
↓	
Excessive tension in outer shoulder muscles	Exercises to improve function of inner shoulder muscles Acupuncture on outer shoulder muscles
↓	↓
Onset of pain in neck and shoulders	Strength training for neck (core)
	↓
	Exercises to balance the whole body Gradually increase loads in training to prepare for returning to sports

*Massage plantar arch: Stimulate the plantar arch by stepping repeatedly on a round oblong object. In Japan, a piece of bamboo is used, but a rolling pin or similarly shaped object can also be used.

● **Table I–2**   Normal and abnormal patterns in scapulohumeral rhythm and pelvic girdle along with lumbago treatment and the preventive measures for shoulder injury. In acupuncture treatment, we must always strive to understand the state of balance in the entire body at the time of treatment. In order to practice this way, in addition to doing orthopedic examinations or range of motion tests in the symptomatic area, we must bear in mind that the symptomatic area is just one part of the whole. One of the characteristics of Oriental medicine is that localized abnormalities are cured by improving the condition of the whole body. Therefore treatment of shoulder injuries has to begin with the treatment of the lower extremities. Likewise, in order to prevent lumbago, fatigue in the lower extremities must be relieved. This is the best way to approach conditioning. As a way of applying this holistic concept of Oriental medicine, we have a simple method of checking the condition of the whole body with movements that stretch various meridians. It is called the Meridian Test method. With this method, the meridian system can be utilized to treat the above-mentioned condition of flatfoot, for example. So instead of just addressing localized muscle pain, we can view the problem as a chain of symptoms that manifest in the whole body as the meridian is stretched (Fig. I–22).

The potential for growth in acupuncture in the field of sports medicine is probably more in the arena of conditioning and improving

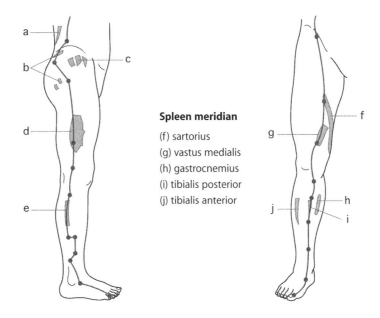

Gallbladder meridian

(a) sacrospinalis
(b) gluteus maximus
(c) gluteus medius
(d) vastus lateralis
(e) peroneus

Spleen meridian

(f) sartorius
(g) vastus medialis
(h) gastrocnemius
(i) tibialis posterior
(j) tibialis anterior

● **Figure I-22**   Meridians and chain of myalgia caused by sinking of the plantar arch

performance than in the treatment of injuries. At the very least, there is a growing recognition in this field of the value of acupuncture for reconditioning. Even if we don't always treat the whole body with acupuncture, we should always aim to improve the condition of the whole body. The essential goal of treatment in Oriental medicine is to create a well-balanced physical condition that facilitates ease in movement, which enables optimal performance. This is exactly how acupuncture should be viewed in the field of sports.

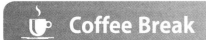 **Coffee Break**

Miraculous Recovery from Back Sprain During a Tennis Match

Moriyama Tomomasa, Professor of the Tsukuba College of Technology

In August 1998, a tennis club in Yugawara of Shizuoka Prefecture held a tennis competition among its members. The men's doubles semifinals were in the seventh game, and it developed into a close match in which their endurance under the blazing sun might decide the winner. The seventh game of the semifinals started as a one-set match for Team A with a 5-2 score. Team A scored 40-30 easily, and was going for the match point. Team B's return ball of Team A's serve touched the net and fell into Team A's court, in front of the forward player. The forward player ran for the ball as fast as he could, but the ball touched the court before he could reach it. The player's momentum tripped him up and he fell over. The score became 40-40: deuce. However, Team A's forward player could not get up, and held his hand on his right hip.

I had been invited to this competition as a trainer and was watching this game. It was clear that the player had twisted his hip as he fell. If the player could not get up, Team A would lose by default. I was called onto the court. I examined the player, and then slowly and deliberately palpated the medial side of his calf on both legs around the acupuncture point KI-9. I quickly needled a point on the right side, which was very tender, and manipulated the needle vigorously. After just a few minutes, the player got up and resumed the game. After that, not only did they score two points in succession and win the semifinal, they kept their momentum and went on to win the finals. Of course, when they took the championship photo, I had to be in it. ●

☕ Coffee Break

Treatment Applying the Meridian Test and the Theory of Biomechanics

Sakuraba Hinata, Licensed Acupuncturist, Student of the Tsukuba College of Technology

Once a young baseball player came to our college clinic complaining of lumbar pain. He was in junior high school in the eighth grade, and was a leading hitter of a senior team in Little League. The doctor who examined him told me, "It's nothing. It's no big deal." Nevertheless, the boy looked to be in too much pain to be standing, and his mother seemed worried. So I immediately performed the Meridian Test ('M-Test'). The movement that caused the most pain was extension of the torso. Aside from this, there were some obvious restrictions in the movement of his lower extremities, but he did not complain of symptoms like pain or fatigue in his legs. Based on my assessment, I treated acupuncture points on the Spleen and Stomach meridians on the torso. This reduced his pain somewhat, but he still had restriction in movement.

From a biomechanical perspective I thought that the loss of elasticity in the muscle groups of the anterior lower extremities due to fatigue may have caused the restriction in the extension of his torso, so I needled additional points on the Spleen and Stomach meridians in the tibialis anterior and the rectus femoris muscles, using the simple insertion[1] technique. The restrictions I observed in his movements were almost gone after needling, and the residual pain in his lumbar area all but disappeared. Neither the patient, who was new to acupuncture, nor his mother could believe that treating his legs could cure his back pain.

In this case, I was able to alleviate pain and restriction in movement by a treatment based on a combination of the M-Test method and my understanding of biomechanics. I have seen many cases like this among athletes in my clinic. The important thing when giving treatment is first to understand the aim of a particular movement in a sport. In baseball, for instance, a pitcher wants to swing his arm faster in order to throw the ball faster. The second thing

---

1. Simple insertion: The needle is inserted to a certain depth and then immediately withdrawn.

we have to understand is how the body needs to move to accomplish the desired aim. There is the macro-view, encompassing the whole movement, as well as the micro-view, that examines each part of the movement in detail by reducing it into movements of individual joints. If one can take both the macro- and micro-views, then it is possible to utilize biomechanics in the treatment. Moreover, when the meridian pathways are applied to each movement, it becomes easy to treat using the M-Test. ●

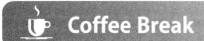

We Don't Need Acupuncturists, Do We?

Sakuraba Hinata, Licensed Acupuncturist, Student of the Tsukuba College of Technology

The other day, I had an opportunity to demonstrate the M-Test method in front of several acupuncturists. As usual, I chose acupuncture points along the course of selected meridians by pressing them to determine their effectiveness, and I concluded by placing several press tacks. After observing my assessment and treatment from start to finish, one acupuncturist who had been licensed for about a year asked a question: "If lay people who don't have acupuncture licenses start to practice the M-Test method using press tacks or acupressure, then there would be no need for acupuncturists, would there?"

This certainly could be true. If anyone could learn to alleviate pain or discomfort associated with movement so simply, then no one would bother seeking out an acupuncturist and pay a high fee to receive treatment. Nevertheless, I look at this way: When we make strenuous physical movements, our muscles have to work, and therefore we cannot avoid muscle fatigue. In the case of athletes, especially, their performance goes on record. Also, they tend to take part in competitions, even to the point of pushing themselves beyond their limits. In times like this, the ability to alleviate pain or discomfort associated with movement would have a great impact on their performance. In many cases, however, fatigue accumulates beyond the body's ability to recover, and athletes are liable to incur injuries. Therefore, it would be ideal if athletes could alleviate pain and discomfort by using the M-Test method on themselves and used it to recover faster from muscle fatigue.

If athletes practice self-care in this way, using press tacks to manage their physical condition on a daily basis as well as during competition, then they are also more likely to seek acupuncture treatment. They will receive acupuncture, which requires specialized knowledge, to deal with health issues beyond the scope of self-care, like chronic muscle tension. For our part, we must establish a comprehensive treatment system so that we can give athletes treatment tailored to their needs. ●

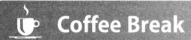

Coffee Break

You Are Fantastic!

Mukaino Yoshito, M.D., Professor of the Faculty of Sports Science, Fukuoka University

"She won a silver metal!" I got a call at my clinic from one of our staff, who had gone to the track field to cheer for an Italian runner competing in the 5000 meter final. It was the summer of 1995, at the Fukuoka Universiade.[1] We had organized a volunteer group calling on acupuncturists, not only from Fukuoka, but from all over Japan. There was much discussion for and against this idea, but we were not officially allowed to run a clinic in the athletes' village. We therefore opened an acupuncture clinic in a hotel room near the athletes' village. The press center was very close to the hotel so our patients could use the shuttle bus between the athletes' village and the press center.

A few days after the opening of our clinic, an Italian track runner named Silvia visited us. She complained that she had not been able to sleep well for a few nights due to the heat and dampness of Fukuoka. She seemed to be desperate and told us that her race would begin in one week. A German doctor, who had come from abroad to study at my laboratory during that time, translated her English for us, and one of our acupuncturists on staff treated her. From the next day on, after seeing Sylvia's spirited practice, lots of Italian athletes came to visit us. As they received treatment, the word "miracle" was heard from many athletes. Sylvia continued to receive treatment every day. One day before the final, she visited our clinic and told us that she placed fifth in the semifinals. We all clapped our hands and encouraged her as we saw her to the door.

According to the phone call I got later, in the final race, Sylvia

---

1. Universiade: An athletic meet of university students from around the world, held every two years. There are summer meets and winter meets.

passed a Japanese runner at the last corner to win the silver medal. When one of our staff saw her running in the finals with the tape of a press tack visible on her body, he muttered, "If only the tape was colored!" (That would have drawn attention to our acupuncture treatments.) I was a bit chagrinned to learn that Sylvia had passed a Japanese runner, but I decided to congratulate her from the bottom of my heart anyway. I believe our entire volunteer staff felt the same way.

The next morning, Silvia visited our clinic with an interpreter. This was despite having run her race late the night before. She showed us her silver medal and said, "Thank you very much. This is the medal I won. I had to show it to you. My flight is today; I'm returning to Italy." I asked her to sign my Universiade T-shirt. She wrote, "You are fantastic! Silvia." We shook hands firmly and exchanged good-byes. It was a hot summer in 1995, when the creation of a nationwide organization for sports acupuncture had just begun. Our efforts then initiated the tradition of organizing teams of volunteer acupuncturists for the annual National Athletic Meet in Japan.[2] ●

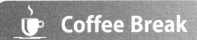

☕ Coffee Break

The Subtle Relationship between Movement and Physical Distortion

Arao Kenji, Teacher at the Fukuoka High School for the Blind

I work at a school for the blind, and am very pleased that sporting events for the visually handicapped have been increasing recently. One of the new events is a game named 'goal ball.' Each team has three players, all of whom are blindfolded, and they stand against their own goal and roll a ball toward the enemy's goal to score points. After a game, or after practicing for a game, right-handed players often suffer severe muscle pain in the right arm and the left posterior leg, especially in the gluteal area, which is used when players step forward. When we performed the M-Test on these players, we found restricted extension in the anterior right arm and restricted extension and flexion in the anterior and posterior left leg.

---

2. National Athletic Meet *(koku-tai)* in Japan: An annual athletic meet held once in the summer and once in the winter, with competition among the urban and rural prefectures of Japan.

The ball that is used in the game is made of rubber, roughly the size of a basketball, and weighing 1.25 kilograms (2.7 pounds). It feels heavy to hold. The player throws this ball with an underarm throw, and the forearm pronates as the hand releases the ball. This puts stress on the anterior arm. I believe this stress can cause restriction in extension of the arm. Also, the player puts all of his or her weight on the forward leg when throwing the ball. This leg is first flexed and then extended. The stress on the anterior and the posterior aspects of this leg can cause a restriction in extension.

When treating this particular presentation, I needle acupuncture points on the Lung and Large Intestine meridians of the arm, as well as the Spleen, Stomach, Kidney, and Bladder meridians, which serves to reduce restriction in extension of the legs. I have seen remarkable improvement with this approach. I noticed something after treating several cases this way: Marked muscle pain or restriction in extension of the leg is not limited to the anterior or posterior aspects, but quite frequently occurs in the lateral aspect as well.

A comment from one of the players gave me a clue to under- standing this phenomenon. People who engage in sports like this probably understand it, but the player said, "If you want to roll a ball with force, you have to step forward, pointing not with your toes, but with the outside of your foot, toward the opposing goal." This could be described as creating a wall toward the goal as you throw the ball. This stance is much more stable, and enables a player to throw the ball fast and powerfully. When you mimic throwing a ball in this manner, you can feel the stress placed on the side of the leg, where the Gallbladder meridian is located.

Knowing how to identify areas with compromised extension after an athletic event gives us a way to determine if the movements are being performed effectively. Just as each sport has its own unique characteristics for causing reduced extension in certain parts of the body, it is also likely that the particular skill or technique of the individual athlete also creates unique restrictions. This case impressed upon me the importance of thorough questioning. I found one other interesting fact while treating the goal ball players. The right-handed player generally has restricted horizontal extension in the medial aspect of the left arm, where the Pericardium meridian is located. This is only a guess, but this restriction in extension could be caused by counterbalancing the load with the arm opposite of the one throwing the ball. The more I use the M-Test, the more curious I have become about the relationship between habitual movements and physical distortions. ●

References

1. Moriyama Tomomasa, *Supotsu ni Okeru Hari Chiryo Ouyo no Rironteki Haikei to Sono Kokakijyo* (Theoretical Basis and Mechanism of Effect for Application of Acupuncture in Sports), *Rinsho Spotsu Igaku* (Japanese Sports Medicine Journal), No. 18 (12), 2001.
2. Mukaino Yoshito, Gerald Kolblinger, and Chen Yong, *Keiraku Tesuto* (Meridian Test), Ishiyaku Shuppan, 1999.

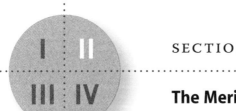

SECTION II

The Meridian Test: Analysis of Movement by Meridians

CHAPTER 1

The Meridian Test and Sensation with Movements

by Honda Tatsuro

Introduction

T HE MOST IMPORTANT CONCERN of every athlete and sports enthusiast is probably how to avoid injury and maintain an optimal state of body and mind in training and competition. Repetition of daily training enables athletes to improve those capabilities that are vital in sporting events including strength, speed, and precision in movement. These capabilities enable athletes to face the challenges of competition in an optimal mental and physical state. It is important to maintain balance and coordination throughout the musculoskeletal system in order to execute effective movements. It is especially important to maintain smooth coordination in the skeletal muscles, which are governed by motor nerves, as well as the joints, which are controlled by skeletal muscles. These coordinated movements involve multiple joints and multiple axes in the body. Where there is pain due to an injury, however, it is impossible to execute the powerful and precise movements that have been developed through daily training. In that situation, an athlete will be unable to draw on his or her full capabilities to perform satisfactorily, and will thus get poor results.

Smooth and coordinated movement throughout the body maintains and improves good performance, and also prevents injuries. The Meridian Test (or 'M-Test') is a valuable method for attaining such smooth movement in the body. It serves as a powerful tool for analyzing abnormalities in movement that span multiple joints and multiple axes. Furthermore, anybody can easily perform this test. The advantage of this method lies in its ability to readily identify areas

45

of restricted movement and obtain specific information about the condition of the body at that point in time.

For instance, one can identify which meridian imbalance is related to fatigue in a part of the body of which the athlete is unaware. In other words, the M-Test makes it possible to make treatment decisions based on an accurate assessment of fatigued areas. In addition, one can quickly, accurately, and easily identify areas of fatigue, which will vary based on the characteristics, positions, and movements of different sports. Moreover, using the M-Test allows one to assess individual differences in areas of fatigue, including those arising from different training routines and incorrect alignment.

In this section I will explain the features of the M-Test and how it assesses specific movements, and the symptoms (discomfort with movement) that are triggered by restrictions in movement.

A. About the Meridian Test

1) FEATURES OF THE MERIDIAN TEST

What kind of an assessment is the M-Test? I will list seven features of this method and present an outline based on my experience.

a. The meridians are stretched to analyze movements.

The M-Test applies the concept of meridians, which is fundamental to acupuncture (Fig. II–1 to II–3). There are twelve regular meridians

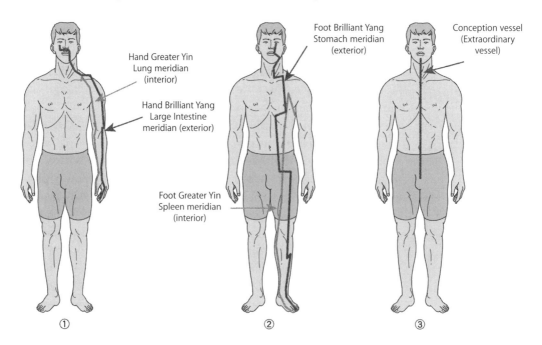

Hand Greater Yin
Lung meridian
(interior)

Hand Brilliant Yang
Large Intestine
meridian (exterior)

Foot Greater Yin
Spleen meridian
(interior)

Foot Brilliant Yang
Stomach meridian
(exterior)

Conception vessel
(Extraordinary
vessel)

①   ②   ③

● **Figure II–1**   Meridians on the anterior aspect

II

and eight extraordinary meridians. The twelve regular meridians are divided into six pairs, and are located bilaterally on the upper and lower extremities. They are also paired into groups based on

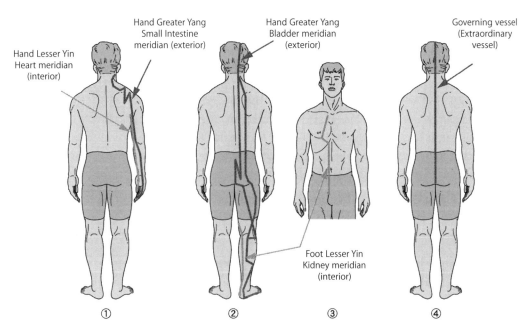

● **Figure II–2** Meridians on the posterior aspect

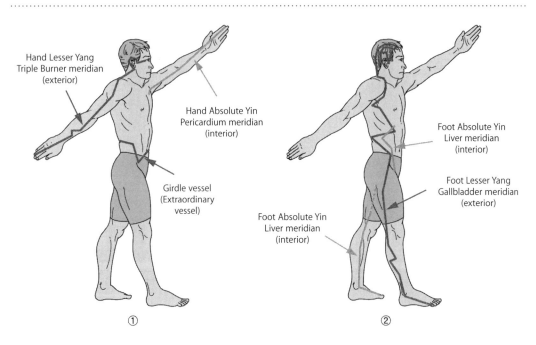

● **Figure II–3** Meridians on the lateral aspect

their name and location (see p. 24). In the M-Test method, one can determine on which meridian the pain or discomfort originates by stretching those aspects of the body on which the meridians are located. For example, if a person has pain in the anterior aspect of the shoulder, stretching movements such as shoulder flexion, extension, horizontal extension, and horizontal flexion are performed (Fig. II–4). If pain is triggered by horizontal extension of the shoulder, for example, then stretching the meridian on the lateral aspect of the arm is viewed as the problem. The meridian located on the lateral aspect of the arm is the Triple Burner meridian, so the diagnosis would be abnormality in the Triple Burner meridian. In this manner, evaluating movements with the M-Test enables one to determine which aspect of the body requires treatment (e.g., the lateral or medial aspect), and the meridians corresponding to that aspect are then treated.

b. The M-Test is composed of complex movements like the basic movements in sports.

The complex movements of athletes in sports as well as the movements in our daily lives all involve multiple joints and multiple axes. When we study the distribution of the meridians on the body (Fig. II–1 to 3) we see that most meridians run vertically from the tips of the toes to the top of the head on the anterior, posterior, and lateral aspects

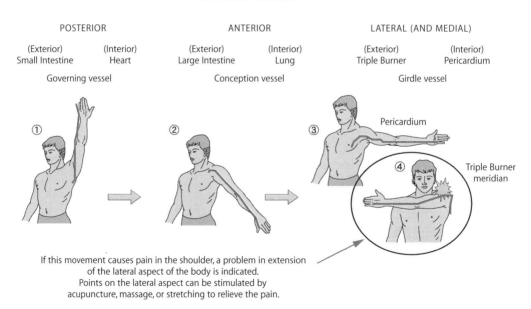

● **Figure II–4**   Stretching meridians to analyze physical movements

ANTERIOR   POSTERIOR   LATERAL (AND MEDIAL)

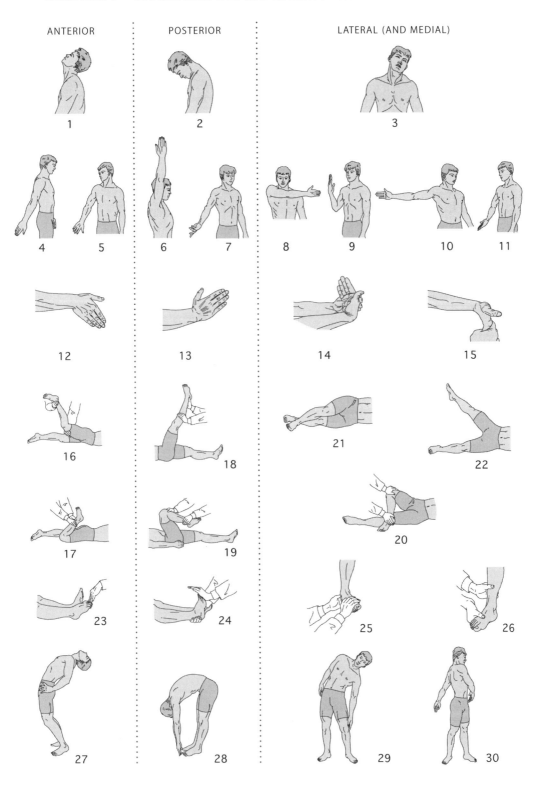

● **Figure II–5**   Standard meridian test stretches for each aspect of the body

of the body. Thus the meridians run across the entire body, including many joints.

The M-Test takes into account the distribution of meridians to evaluate movements of the body in relation to its three aspects: anterior, posterior, and lateral. The M-Test consists of thirty simple movements, shown in Figure II–5. These movements serve as the foundation for the more complex movements that we make in our daily lives, as well as in sports. Movements in sports, especially, can be understood as being composed of simple basic motions that are combined in complex ways. Figure II–6 shows the example of a running form in a track race. Running is a basic movement in many types of sports. When we break down the running form by dividing it into movements in each part of the body, we find that it is composed of simple, basic movements that are included in the M-Test. We can examine the basic movements that make up the more complex movements, and determine whether each one is executed smoothly. We should be able to bring the movements in sports closer to an ideal form by identifying and treating any restrictions in the basic movements.

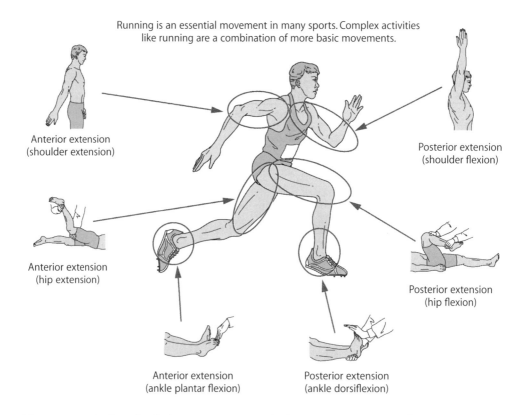

Running is an essential movement in many sports. Complex activities like running are a combination of more basic movements.

Anterior extension
(shoulder extension)

Posterior extension
(shoulder flexion)

Anterior extension
(hip extension)

Posterior extension
(hip flexion)

Anterior extension
(ankle plantar flexion)

Posterior extension
(ankle dorsiflexion)

● **Figure II–6**   M-Test checks basic movements which comprise more complex movements

In addition to the thirty simple movements of the M-Test, there are of course a number of variations. Examples of variations for the test with the shoulder in horizontal flexion are shown in Figure II–7. In the first variation, the arm is rotated laterally with the elbow flexed, and in the second variation, the arm is rotated medially with the elbow flexed. These movements are each similar to the beginning and end of a throwing motion essential to sports like baseball. They also somewhat resemble the motion of combing the hair or fastening a belt. These tests are often positive for conditions like periarthritis or frozen shoulder. Horizontal flexion of the shoulder coupled with lateral rotation torques the superior aspect of the shoulder and also stretches the anterior aspect of the upper arm. Likewise, horizontal flexion of the shoulder with medial rotation torques the inferior aspect of the shoulder and also stretches the posterior aspect of the upper arm.

Extension of posterior aspect   Extension of anterior aspect

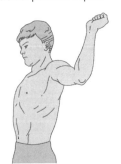 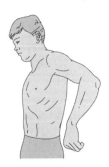

Horizontal flexion of shoulder   Horizontal extension of shoulder
(elbow in flexion)   (elbow in flexion)

● **Figure II–7** Shoulder movements affecting anterior and posterior aspects

c. Both the athlete and the trainer or therapist can verify restrictions and improvements in movement.

Orthopedic and neurological tests are performed to determine the affected parts and the cause of pain. The aim of Meridian Testing is not only to find pain, but also to detect sensations such as tightness, discomfort, and fatigue. Furthermore, we look for differences between the right and left sides when doing the same movement in the arms and legs. Usually an athlete is unaware of minor restrictions in movement when he or she is able to perform daily activities and carry on their training without a problem. By means of the M-Test, however, an athlete may become aware of the existence of a restriction in movement for the first time. Furthermore, the person performing the tests can confirm the tension in the muscles and the decrease in the range of motion (ROM).

When athletes use the M-Test to assess their own physical condition, we can apply the results of their self-administered M-Test to their daily training and stretching routines and thereby prevent injury. We can also keep track of the constantly changing state of their muscles and ROMs with the accumulation of fatigue, and put this information to use in our treatment.

d. The M-Test can make stretching exercises and sports massage more effective.

Stretching before the commencement of exercise is a common practice even among those who are not athletes as such. Most people, however, routinely repeat the same stretching exercises. In Japan, for example, it is still common to see everyone in a physical education class or on a sports team do the same stretching exercises together, or exchanging whole body massages, and devoting a lot of time to this. However, the area of the body where thorough stretching or massage is needed differs according to the sport, and depends on its demands. Even within the same sport, different playing positions may require stretching or massaging of different areas of the body. It is also possible that, based on the athlete's codition, the areas and types of stretching and massage need to be changed every day. The aim of stretching and massage essentially is to take the kinks out of muscles, promote circulation, and facilitate smooth movement. If the physical condition of athletes was always the same, then the stretching and massage could always be the same; but this is almost never the case. What is usually required is thorough stretching or massage of the areas that need it the most, according to the athlete's physical condition.

The M-Test enables us to identify where the restrictions to stretching exist (in either the anterior, posterior, or lateral aspect of the body) in relation to the perceived problems in movement. In this method we learn which meridians are involved and which movements need to be improved. One way is to have the athlete quickly go through the movements of the M-Test on his own, and then ask him to carefully stretch (or give him a massage) focusing just on the muscles in the area with tension or discomfort. Figure II–8 provides some examples of stretching exercises that are beneficial for restrictions identified by the M-Test in the lateral aspect of the body. The treatment method, and the amount of stimulation, can be determined based on the situation. As a rule, the most effective level of stimulation for relieving muscle tension is low intensity work that feels pleasant to the athlete. Therefore, especially after a workout, a comfortable level of stimulation is recommended.

M-TEST POSITIVE SIGNS   STRETCHES (EXAMPLES)

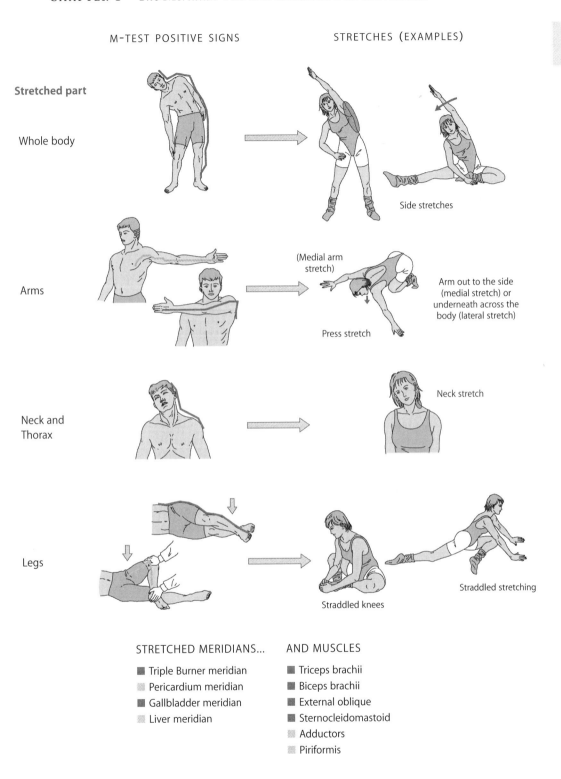

Stretched part

Whole body

Side stretches

Arms

(Medial arm stretch)

Press stretch

Arm out to the side (medial stretch) or underneath across the body (lateral stretch)

Neck and Thorax

Neck stretch

Legs

Straddled knees

Straddled stretching

STRETCHED MERIDIANS...   AND MUSCLES

- Triple Burner meridian
- Pericardium meridian
- Gallbladder meridian
- Liver meridian

- Triceps brachii
- Biceps brachii
- External oblique
- Sternocleidomastoid
- Adductors
- Piriformis

● **Figure II–8**   Example of stretching exercises for restricted movements (lateral aspects)

e. The M-Test can be used not only for examination and assessment of sports injuries, but also for conditioning of the athlete.

Nowadays, athletes regard conditioning to be just as important as training. We have to take up the challenge to integrate conditioning—including stretching, massage, and nutrition, as well as the mental aspect—into the training of athletes. The benefit of applying the M-Test is that the intensity of the training regimen and the stretching or massage can be modified to suit an athlete at a specific point in time. This makes it possible to provide more effective training, stretching, and massage. An athlete's physical condition differs from day to day, and this difference is reflected in the results of the M-Test. For instance, not just athletes, but everybody occasionally experiences feelings of fatigue and a resulting loss of concentration and motivation. For best results, one can undertake training based on the results of the M-Test, and take into account that the condition of some part of the body is not the same as usual. In certain cases, we have to consider whether the training program should be modified. Also, appropriate modalities of conditioning, such as stretching and massage, can be applied effectively by targeting the fatigued areas.

f. Since the movements in the M-Test are similar to those in orthopedic tests, doctors and physical therapists find it easy to understand, and athletes can therefore be cared for by a medical team.

Orthopedic tests are very useful for determining if there is an injury, trauma, or impediment in the body, and to identify the location of the lesion. Several of the movements assessed in the M-Test are the same as those tested by orthopedic and neurological tests. For example, the movements for the SLR (straight leg raising) test and the Fabere Patrick test, which are typically performed when evaluating cases of low back pain, are part of the M-Test. These movements are shown in illustrations 18 and 20 of Figure II–5. In the M-Test, however, in addition to pain, practitioners also assess sensations of tightness and discomfort, as well as differences between the right and left sides.

I work with physical therapists as a trainer looking after athletes. When an athlete comes to us complaining of low back pain, the physical therapist first performs the orthopedic tests, such as the Patrick test. When the Patrick test triggers pain, we suspect an abnormality in the hip or sacroiliac joint. In the M-Test, on the other hand, pain triggered by the Patrick test indicates inadequate extension in the medial aspect of the leg. For this condition, treatment on the medial and lateral aspects of the leg (the Liver and Gallbladder meridians) is suggested, and indurations (abnormally tight areas or nodules) in the muscles or skin of those areas are treated. Since the M-

Test and the orthopedic tests check certain movements in common, the findings can be used for both approaches. Some Western medical practitioners, including physicians, have had an issue with Oriental medicine because it is difficult to understand. The use of the M-Test helps remove this obstacle, and enables acupuncturists to work side by side with Western medical practitioners as members of a medical team.

2.) THE THIRTY MOVEMENTS OF THE MERIDIAN TEST

The M-Test is comprised of movements that extend or stretch tissues along the twelve regular meridians. These thirty basic movements are shown in Figure II–5. Some of these movements also stretch tissues along the extraordinary meridians, including the Conception vessel and Governing vessel. The thirty movements are classified into anterior, posterior, and lateral (including medial) aspects of the body corresponding to the location of the meridians. The movements in the M-Test are configured so that the relationship between a particular extension or stretch and specific meridians can be easily identified. The movements of the M-Test include gross movements down to very small movements of the wrist and ankle. In this way, the M-Test enables us to check restrictions in every part of the body, including the whole body, neck, torso, arms, and legs.

Table II–1 describes the basic movements of the M-Test and the areas of the body that each of these movements stretch. Please refer to this table as you read the following sections: a) the anterior meridians and their associated test movements; b) the posterior meridians and their associated test movements; and c) the lateral (and medial) meridians and their associated test movements.

a. Anterior meridians and their associated test movements

On the anterior aspect of the body, the meridians on the arm are the Lung and Large Intestine meridians, the meridians on the leg are the Spleen and Stomach meridians, and the Conception vessel lies on the midline of the torso (see Fig. II–1). Movements that extend the anterior aspect of the body are said to stretch these meridians (see Fig. II–5, left column). When any of these movements causes pain or resistance, these are the primary meridians to treat.

The kicking motion in soccer requires a strong and swift forward movement of the leg. When this is done repeatedly, the muscles in the anterior aspect of the leg, including the quadriceps femoris, sartorius, and tibialis anterior, are prone to fatigue. Movements of the anterior aspect of the leg are compromised when fatigue accumulates in these muscles. In this case, positive signs are obtained when M-Test movements are performed for the anterior aspect of the leg.

No. in Fig. II–5	M-Test movements	Areas stretched
ANTERIOR		
1	Neck extension	Anterior neck and chest
4	Shoulder extension with arm extended	Arm and chest
5	Elbow pronation	Arm around anterior aspect of elbow
12	Wrist ulnar flexion	Radial wrist and forearm
16	Prone hip extension with knee extended	Anterior thigh and inguinal region (same as FNS test*)
17	Prone knee flexion	Knee, anterior thigh, and inguinal region
23	Supine plantar flexion	Anterior ankle and lower leg
27	Standing torso extension	Anterior neck down to anterior legs
POSTERIOR		
2	Neck flexion	Occipital region to upper back
6	Shoulder flexion with arm extended	Lateral arm and scapula
7	Elbow supination	Arm around posterior aspect of elbow
13	Wrist radial flexion	Ulnar wrist and forearm
18	Supine hip flexion with knee extended	Posterior lower extremity (same as SLR test*)
19	Supine hip flexion with knee flexed	Posterior thigh to gluteal region
24	Supine dorsiflexion	Posterior ankle and lower leg
28	Standing torso flexion	Posterior neck down to posterior legs
LATERAL		
3	Neck lateral flexion	Lateral neck to shoulder
8	Horizontal extension of shoulder with arm extended	Posterior arm to medial scapula
9	Elbow flexion	Elbow to posterior arm
10	Horizontal flexion of shoulder with arm extended	Medial arm to chest
11	Elbow extension	Medial aspect of arm
14	Wrist flexion	Posterior aspect of wrist & forearm
15	Wrist extension	Anterior aspect of wrist & forearm
20	Lateral rotation of hip with knee flexed	Medial thigh and inguinal region (same as Patrick test*)
21	Supine hip adduction	Lateral aspect of leg and hip
22	Supine hip abduction	Medial leg and inguinal region
25	Ankle supination	Lateral aspect of foot and lower leg
26	Ankle pronation	Medial aspect of foot and lower leg
29	Sidebend torso	Lateral aspect of torso and leg
30	Twist torso	Lateral torso centered around waist

● **Table II–1**   M-Test movements and extended sections (see Figure II–5)

FNS test = Femoral nerve stretch test: an orthopedic exam for femoral nerve impingement.
SLR test = Straight leg raising test: an orthopedic exam for sciatica.
Patrick test = Fabere Patrick test: an orthopedic exam for hip joint lesions.

II

b. Posterior meridians and their associated test movements

On the anterior aspect of the body, the meridians on the arm are the Heart and Small Intestine meridians, the meridians on the leg are the Kidney and the Bladder meridians, and the Governing vessel is on the midline of the torso (see Fig. II–2). Movements that extend the posterior aspect of the body are said to stretch these meridians (see Fig. II–5, center column). An exception, however, is the upper portion of the Kidney meridian, because it lies on the anterior aspect of the torso. When any of these movements causes an abnormal sensation, such as pain or resistance, these are the primary meridians to treat.

Running in track and field events requires vigorous stepping motions, and in order to run fast, the feet must hit the ground hard. The muscles on the posterior aspect of the leg, such as the triceps surae and hamstrings, receive a considerable impact when the heels hit the ground in this manner. Thus fatigue accumulates in these muscles; moreover, this can lead to injuries, such as torn muscles. When we perform the M-Test on athletes who run, we tend to get findings analogous to the above situation, and there are usually problems in movements that stretch the posterior aspect of the legs.

c. Lateral (and medial) meridians and their associated test movements

In addition to the anterior and posterior aspects, there is also the lateral aspect of the body, which includes the medial aspect in the M-Test. On the arms, the Pericardium meridian is located on the medial aspect and the Triple Burner meridian on the lateral aspect. On the legs, the Liver meridian is located on the medial aspect and the Gallbladder meridian on the lateral aspect. In addition, the Girdle vessel, an Extraordinary meridian, encircles the torso at the waist (see Fig. II–3). Movements that extend the lateral (or medial) aspect of the body are said to stretch these meridians (see Fig. II–5, right column). When any of these movements causes abnormal sensations, such as pain or resistance, these are the primary meridians to treat.

Soccer and basketball players (among others) are required to make sudden movements to the left or right, in response to movements by their opponents. So they engage in rapid and forceful dodging and shifting of direction. These players tend to stress the muscles in the medial and lateral aspects of the legs, such as the tensor fasciae latae, iliotibial tract, and adductor muscles, and these muscles tend to become fatigued. This tendency is seen in confrontational sports like soccer and basketball because the situation changes moment to moment and the players are never sure which movement they are going to make. When these athletes experience fatigue in the lateral or medial aspect of the legs, the M-Test movements stretching the lateral and medial aspects tend to show up positive.

d. What constitutes a positive finding in the M-Test?

In the M-Test the criteria for a positive finding are subjective sensations such as discomfort, heaviness, tension, and pain associated with a particular movement. We assess the condition of the body at the time by noting which of the thirty test movements causes abnormal sensations. For instance, if there is a restriction in the hip abduction movement (test movement 20: Patrick test), we can determine whether the restriction is accompanied by discomfort or pain. Sometimes the ROM in the hips is clearly limited, or there is a marked difference between the ROM in the left hip and the right hip, but there is no abnormal sensation associated with the test. This should also be viewed as a positive finding. What the practitioner feels can also constitute a positive finding. For instance, when hip flexion is performed passively, any resistance felt by the practitioner, as well as right/left differences in the places where resistance is felt, is relevant to the assessment.

B. The Relationships among Restricted Motion, Fatigue, and Injury

1) THE RELATIONSHIP BETWEEN FATIGUE AND INJURY IN SPORTS

The occurrence of injuries in sports is closely related to the deterioration in the quality of movements due to overuse. Fatigue in the skeletal muscles is one of the factors causing deterioration in the quality of movement. According to a survey of students in the Department of Sports and Health Science at Fukuoka University, about 70 percent of students believed the cause of sports injuries is fatigue from training. Therefore, for the athletes and sports lovers, countermeasures against muscle fatigue are important also from the standpoint of preventing injury. It is not that easy, however, to pinpoint the location or the extent of fatigue because the muscles and the parts of the body used differ from event to event and depend on the nature of the event. Moreover, the part of the body that becomes fatigued can differ from athlete to athlete because of abnormal alignment, the training regimen, and the position played.

Almost all fatigue in the skeletal muscles from sports activity usually resolves when the athlete gets some rest. Muscle fatigue accumulates, however, when this fatigue is not resolved completely and this affects the quality of movement and the ROM. In other words, compared to the normal condition of the athlete, the quality of movement is compromised. When an athlete trains in this condition (with significant restrictions in movement) it creates a vicious cycle of fatigue spreading to other parts of the body. Furthermore, engaging in competition in this condition with compromised movements compounds the stress on certain parts of the body, and this can lead to an injury. This is why it is important to take countermeasures to relieve fatigue in the early stage.

2) Progress from fatigue to injury

The mechanism leading from fatigue to injury is complex and difficult to explain in a just few words. Nevertheless, by treating athletes using the M-Test, we can visualize the process by which fatigue leads to an injury by correlating the positive findings of the M-Test with information gathered from questioning (Fig. II–9).

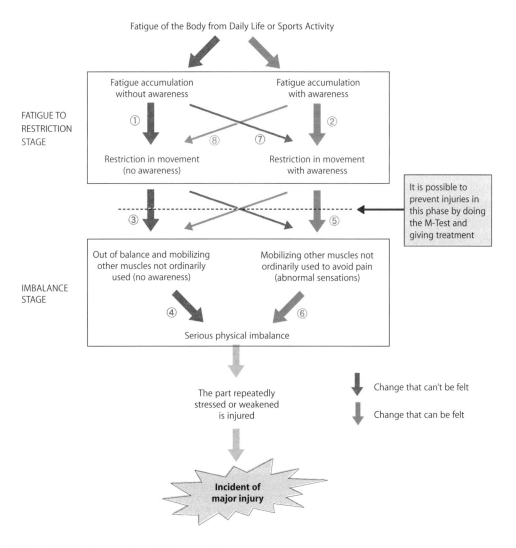

● **Figure II–9**   Process from fatigue to injury

a. Fatigue to restriction stage (top of Fig. II–9)

There are two possible situations with physical fatigue that is caused by and accumulates from sports or daily activities. In the first case, one is aware of the fatigue, and in the second case, one is not. We will examine fatigue by dividing it into these two categories. 'Fatigue without awareness' is fatigue that is not felt by the athlete even if there is restriction in movement caused by the fatigue (① in the figure). 'Fatigue with awareness,' on the other hand, usually occurs when the amount of fatigue is considerably greater and the athlete is aware of compromised movement or a decline in performance (② in the figure). An athlete can prevent injury if he or she does the M-Test to discover which movements are compromised and takes steps to correct these while still in the 'fatigue to restriction' stage.

b. Imbalance stage (middle of Fig. II–9)

When 'fatigue without awareness' gradually accumulates, restrictions in movement increase in proportion to the amount of fatigue (③ in the figure). As a result, the body is in a state of imbalance, and one unconsciously starts to employ other parts of the body to perform certain movements. An even greater state of physical imbalance is created as one continues to exercise or play in this condition, and the weak part of the body or the area under repetitive stress becomes damaged and prone to injury (④ in the figure). This progression from fatigue to injury is described, based on one clinical case, in Figure II–10.

 On the other hand, it is not normal even when one can feel the fatigue and is aware of a restriction in movement. In many cases the muscles will experience abnormal sensations, such as a feeling of tension or pain (⑤ in the figure). For example, when there is pain and an athlete continues to train under this condition of pain and probable muscle strain, he or she will move in such as way as to avoid the pain. Thus other parts of the body, or even the other side of the body, that is normally not used for the movement are employed. This sets up a vicious cycle, which creates even more serious imbalances and damages the weak part or the area under repetitive stress (⑥ in the figure).

 One commonly seen example of this is in people with ankle sprain by inversion. After a while, the fatigue in the tibialis anterior or the peroneus muscle on the injured side grows worse. This commonly leads to pain in the opposite ankle or knee due to overcompensation.

c. Other patterns (top of Fig. II–9)

There are other atypical patterns of progress from fatigue to injury, such as suddenly feeling a decline in the quality of movement after accumulating fatigue that one is unaware of (⑦ in the figure).

Conversely, one can be aware of considerable fatigue in the body, but unaware of a decline in the quality of movement, which gradually progresses to restriction in movement. (⑧ in the figure). In either case, it is possible that a large imbalance can be created that will lead to an injury. Such atypical patterns include cases where athletes hit a slump after overtraining because their form gradually deteriorated without their awareness.

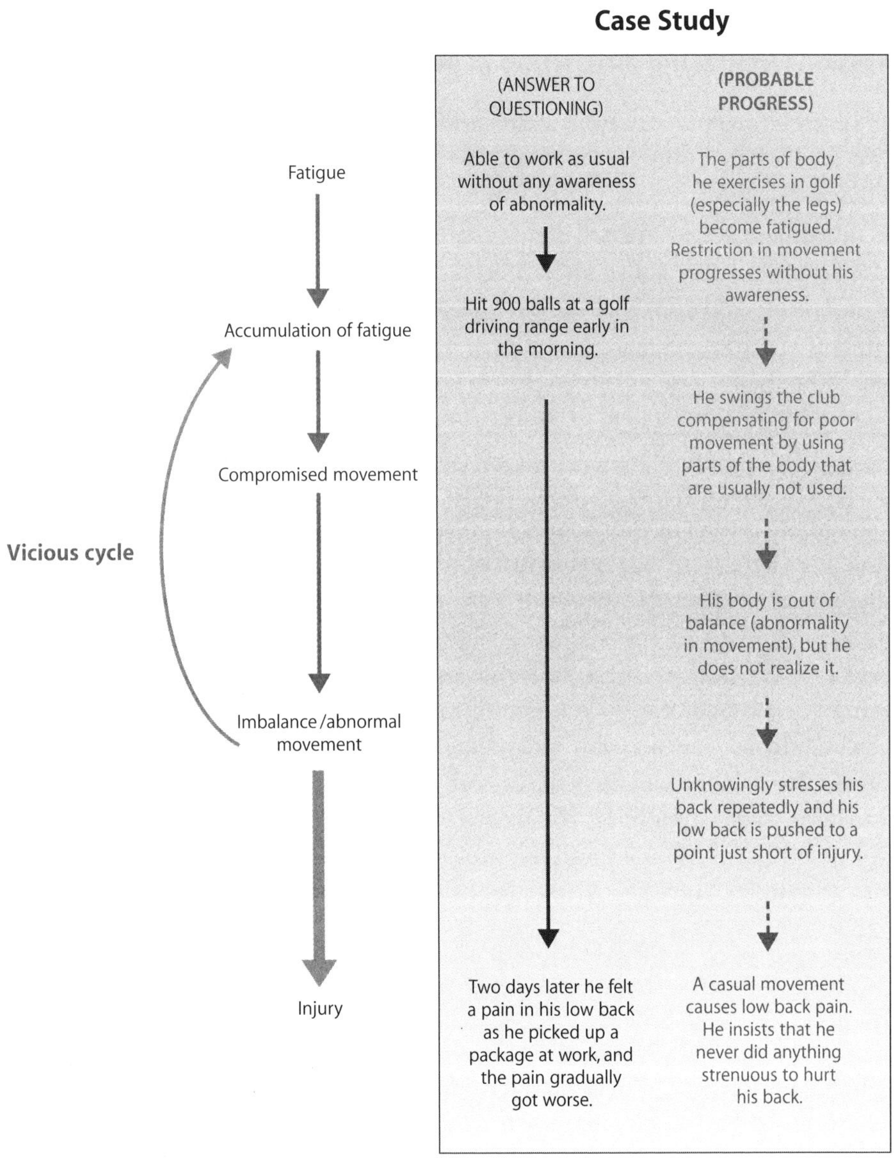

Case Study

	(ANSWER TO QUESTIONING)	(PROBABLE PROGRESS)
Fatigue	Able to work as usual without any awareness of abnormality.	The parts of body he exercises in golf (especially the legs) become fatigued. Restriction in movement progresses without his awareness.
Accumulation of fatigue	Hit 900 balls at a golf driving range early in the morning.	
Compromised movement		He swings the club compensating for poor movement by using parts of the body that are usually not used.
Vicious cycle		His body is out of balance (abnormality in movement), but he does not realize it.
Imbalance/abnormal movement		Unknowingly stresses his back repeatedly and his low back is pushed to a point just short of injury.
Injury	Two days later he felt a pain in his low back as he picked up a package at work, and the pain gradually got worse.	A casual movement causes low back pain. He insists that he never did anything strenuous to hurt his back.

● **Figure II–10**   A case study of progress from fatigue to injury

The M-Test is a tool that allows athletes and sports enthusiasts to assess their physical condition based on the subjective sensations of different movements, using the felt sense of being in good condition as the standard. This enables us to determine at a very early stage if any restrictions in movement have developed, and how much a particular movement is compromised, compared to when the athlete is in top form. In addition to preventing injuries, this assessment can prevent a slump or help an athlete find a way out of a slump.

C. Sensations Indicating Restriction in Movement

Detecting restrictions in movement at an early stage to reduce fatigue in training is useful for conditioning as well as the prevention of injury. Identifying restrictions in movement is also essential for effectively treating an athlete following an injury. The criteria for detecting restrictions in the early stage include sensations like discomfort, heaviness, tension, and pain that are elicited by a series of stretching movements. I call these 'kinetic sensations.' These kinetic sensations enable us to easily grasp abnormalities in the meridians (movement) at a given point in time. In other words, by using the M-Test, we can understand the functional condition of the entire body in detail and take countermeasures to correct abnormalities. In rare cases a kinetic sensation cannot be elicited even when the ROM of a joint is reduced and there is an obvious restriction in movement, or even when there is a big difference between right and left legs doing the same movement. Also, there are cases where no kinetic sensation is felt when a test movement is performed passively, even though the amount of resistance felt by the examiner indicates a restriction in movement. In such cases, the judgment of the examiner takes precedence. The subject will be able to feel the difference (kinetic sensation) after some treatment. In this way, the M-Test is more effective when the sensations of both the subject and the examiner are taken into account as movements are performed to assess the quality of movement.

References

1. Mukaino Yoshito, et al., "The Meridian Test: A new method of defining effective meridians for the treatment of painful disorders of the neck by acupuncture." Proceedings of the FISU/CESU Conference, the 18th Universiade Fukuoka, p. 198-199, 1995.
2. Mukaino Yoshito, Gerald Kolblinger, and Chen Yong, *Keiraku Tesuto* (Meridian Test), Ishiyaku Shuppan, 1999.

3. Honda Tatsuo, *Keiraku Tesuto o Mochi-ita Hari Chiryo* (Acupuncture Treatment Applying the Meridian Test) *Rinsho Spotsu Igaku* (Japanese Sports Medicine Journal), no. 18: 1383–1388, 2001.

4. Mukaino Yoshito, *Keiraku Tesuto ni Yoru Shindan to Hari Chiryo* (Diagnosis and Acupunture Treatment Using the Meridian Test), Ishiyaku Shuppan, 2002.

5. *Mukaino Yoshito, Supotsu ni Okeru Shinkyu Ouyo no Rironteki Haikei to Sono Kokakijyo* (The Theoretical Basis and Mechanism of Effect for Application of Acupuncture in Sports), *Rinsho Spotsu Igaku* (Japanese Sports Medicine Journal) no. 17: 1033–1042, 2000.

CHAPTER 2

2

Muscles Involved in the Meridian Test

by Kitaoka Yuko

Introduction

There are thee planes of movement in the body. They are the sagittal plane, the frontal or coronal plane, and the transverse plane (Fig. II–11). The movements in sports consist of multiple combinations of movement in these three planes. The complexity of combinations in planes of movement can be understood easily when we compare the figures in Figure II–12. The figure on the left shows the simple movement in abdominal muscle building (sit-ups) and the figure on the right shows the complex movement of batting in baseball. In other words, movements in sports involve multiple joints and multiple axes, as well as multiple planes. Particularly in sports, there is a complex combination of movements through various planes, and many sports involve sequences of such combinations. If one ignores this characteristic of movements in training, optimal results of training cannot be demonstrated in the game.

Sometimes conditioning is not appropriate due to a lack of understanding about the characteristics of movements in the sport. In order to avoid such an oversight, instead of focusing on individual muscles in training, all movements in sports must be seen as a sequence of movements *involving many muscles*. With this understanding, training can be done taking into consideration the characteristics of movements in each event, as well as the complexity of these movements involving multiple joints, multiple axes, and multiple planes. The training regimen can be designed to fit the particular movement patterns. In other words, functional training is what is required. The

65

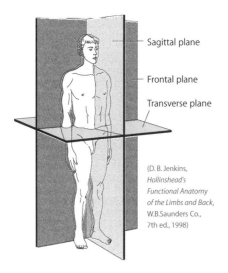

Sagittal plane

Frontal plane

Transverse plane

(D. B. Jenkins, *Hollinshead's Functional Anatomy of the Limbs and Back*, W.B.Saunders Co., 7th ed., 1998)

● **Figure II–11**   Planes of movement

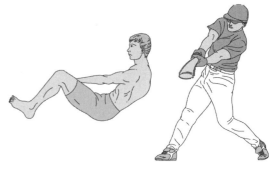

In a sit-up, the pelvis is anchored to the floor and movements are limited to the sagittal plane. The pelvic girdle is not anchored as abdominal muscles are used in sports like tennis or baseball. Thus movement of the torso is a complex combination in all three planes.

● **Figure II–12**   Differences in use of abdominal muscles in simple exercise and in playing sports

issue of fatigue and injury in sports must also be viewed from this perspective.

Beyond the conventional approach, which is focused on the movement and function of individual joints, the M-Test allows us to analyze movements from the perspective of multiple joints, multiple axes, and multiple planes. In this way, the M-Test enables us to more accurately assess how fatigue and injury affect the ability to engage in sports. Furthermore, by appropriately treating any abnormality in movement with acupuncture or stretching, we can restore the linkage of smooth movement in individual joints. In this way, the M-Test enables athletes to execute movements that are closer to the ideal. This in turn improves their performance, reduces the accumulation of fatigue, and prevents injuries.

In this section I will discuss the muscles that are involved in each one of the movements of the M-Test and their functions.

A. The Skeletal Muscles

1) Illustrations of the Skeletal Muscles

There are about 650 skeletal muscles in the human body. Since almost all of these muscles are on both sides the body, we can learn the names of all the skeletal muscles by memorizing about 300 names. First, I will present the primary surface muscles in the anterior, posterior, medial, and lateral aspects (see Fig. II 13–15). The muscles of the forearm, which are involved in the movement of the wrist joint in particular, are composed of many small muscles. For this reason, I

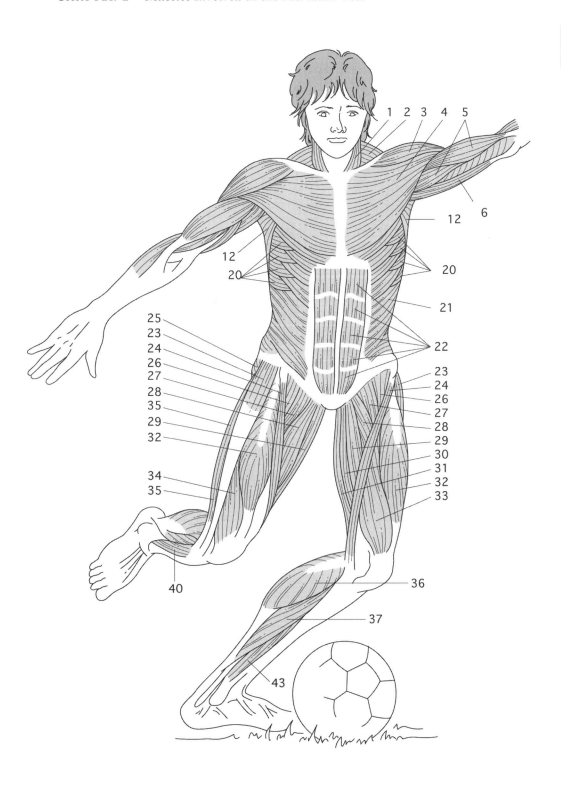

● **Figure II–13**   Superficial muscles of anterior aspect

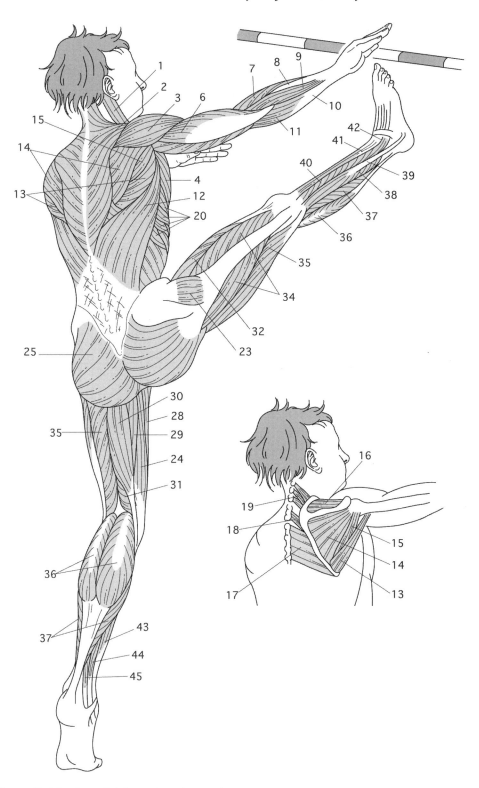

● **Figure II–14**   Superficial muscles of posterior aspect

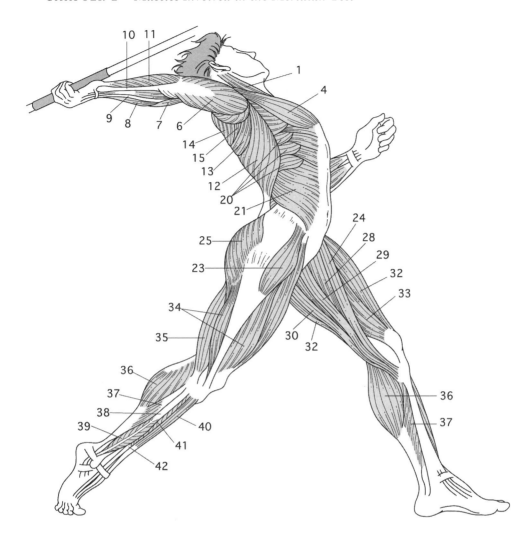

● **Figure II–15**   Superficial muscles of lateral aspect

1 Sternocleidomastoid
2 Trapezius
3 Deltoid
4 Pectoralis major
5 Biceps brachii
6 Triceps brachii
7 Brachioradialis
8 Extensor carpi radialis longus and brevis
9 Extensor digitorum communis
10 Extensor carpi ulnaris
11 Flexor carpi ulnaris
12 Latissimus dorsi
13 Teres major
14 Infraspinatus
15 Teres minor

16 Supraspinatus
17 Rhomboid major
18 Rhomboid minor
19 Levator scapulae
20 Serratus anterior
21 External oblique
22 Rectus abdominis
23 Tensor fasciae latae
24 Sartorius
25 Gluteus maximus
26 Iliopsoas
27 Pectineus
28 Adductor magnus
29 Gracilis
30 Semitendinosus

31 Semimembranosus
32 Rectus femoris
33 Vastus medialis
34 Vastus lateralis
35 Biceps femoris
36 Gastrocnemius
37 Soleus
38 Peroneus longus
39 Peroneus brevis
40 Tibialis anterior
41 Extensor hallucis longus
42 Extensor digitorum longus
43 Tibialis posterior
44 Flexor hallucis longus
45 Flexor digitorum longus

(Figures on pages 67–69 are from Wirhed, R., *Athletic Ability and Anatomy of Motion*, 3rd ed., Mosby, 2006.)

will present the forearm muscles of wrist flexion by cross section in three layers: surface, middle, and deep. Likewise the muscles of wrist extension are shown in two layers: surface and deep. Figure II–16 shows the cross section of the forearm.

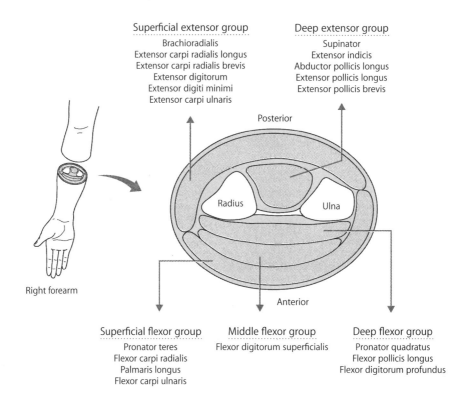

Superficial extensor group
Brachioradialis
Extensor carpi radialis longus
Extensor carpi radialis brevis
Extensor digitorum
Extensor digiti minimi
Extensor carpi ulnaris

Deep extensor group
Supinator
Extensor indicis
Abductor pollicis longus
Extensor pollicis longus
Extensor pollicis brevis

Posterior

Radius   Ulna

Right forearm

Anterior

Superficial flexor group
Pronator teres
Flexor carpi radialis
Palmaris longus
Flexor carpi ulnaris

Middle flexor group
Flexor digitorum superficialis

Deep flexor group
Pronator quadratus
Flexor pollicis longus
Flexor digitorum profundus

● **Figure II–16**   Muscles of the forearm: cross-sectional grouping

2) Functions of the Muscles

Most movement in the body occurs through the action of the joints. The primary motivating components of the joints are the muscles. The muscles constitute about 40 percent of the entire weight of the body. Muscles not only enable locomotion, but also serve the functions of maintaining posture as well as producing body heat.

a. Locomotion

The muscles contract and relax with signals from the brain. The contraction of skeletal muscles creates the movement in joints.

b. Production of body heat

All cells in the body produce heat in the process of energy metabolism. Muscles are a primary source of heat production.

c. Maintaining posture

The skeletal system creates a support structure for the body, and the skeletal muscles maintain this structure. Also, the skeletal muscles serve a role in stabilizing and keeping joints stationary so that other parts can move.

3) MUSCLES AND MOVEMENT

a. The origin and insertion of muscles

All muscles have tendons on each end, and the tendons attach to bones and enable movement in the joints, which connect the bones. Almost all skeletal muscles cross over joints and attach to the bones on either side. When the muscle contracts, the bone on one side of the joint moves closer to the bone on the other side. This produces movement in the joint. Generally, one bone remains stationary and only the bone on the other side of the joint moves to create movement. The site where the tendon attaches to the stationary bone is called the origin of the muscle, and the site where the tendon attaches on the moving bone is called the insertion (Fig. II–17). All 650 skeletal muscles have origins and insertions. Figure II–18 shows a muscle of the upper arm (brachialis), which is a flexor of the elbow joint, along with its origin and insertion. If you know which muscle originates and inserts on which bones (crossing over which joint), then you know the joint that the muscle moves as a matter of course.

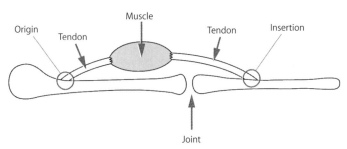

● **Figure II–17**   Basic model of a muscle

b. Primary movers, antagonists, synergists, and stabilizers (position fixers)

Movement in joints is created by two or more muscles working together in concert. The antagonists are the muscles located on the opposite side of the bones from the primary movers. They relax or extend as the primary movers contract. Synergists are muscles that assist the primary movers. The stabilizers or position fixers are

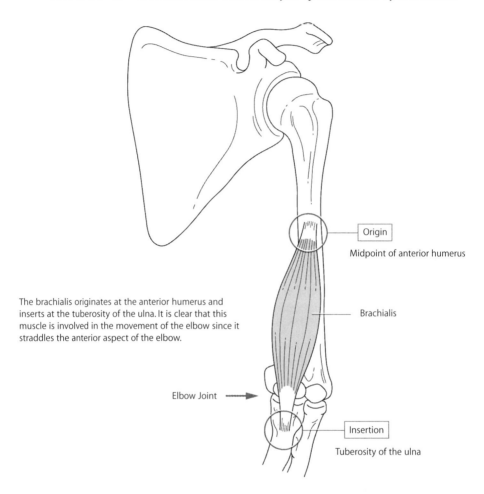

The brachialis originates at the anterior humerus and inserts at the tuberosity of the ulna. It is clear that this muscle is involved in the movement of the elbow since it straddles the anterior aspect of the elbow.

Origin
Midpoint of anterior humerus

Brachialis

Elbow Joint

Insertion
Tuberosity of the ulna

● **Figure II–18**   Origin, insertion, and function of the brachialis muscle

muscles that serve to stabilize the joint during movement. In this way, many muscles work together to enable smooth motion in a single body movement.

The muscles that contract to generate movement in the joint are the primary movers. The muscles located on the opposite side of the joint are the antagonists. The primary movers and the antagonists switch their roles when a joint movement is reversed. For example, when the hamstrings (biceps femoris, semitendinosus, and semimembranosus) contract, the calf moves backward and the knee joint flexes. To allow this movement, the quadriceps muscles on the opposite side (rectus femoris, vastus lateralis, vastus medialis, and vastus medialis) must stretch. In this movement, the hamstrings are the primary mover, and the quadriceps are the antagonist. Conversely, to produce the opposite movement (flexion of the hip and extension of the knee) the quadriceps must contract and the hamstrings must extend. In this movement, the quadriceps are the primary mover and the hamstring is the antagonist. Figure II–19 shows the relationship of the primary mover and the antagonist in elbow flexion.

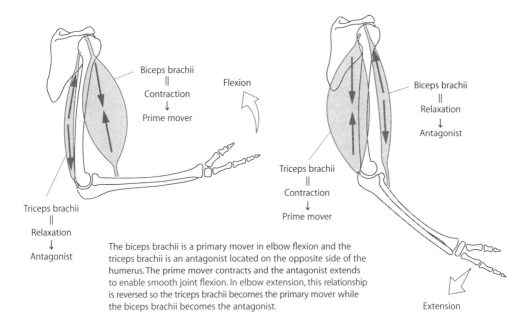

Biceps brachii
‖
Contraction
↓
Prime mover

Flexion

Biceps brachii
‖
Relaxation
↓
Antagonist

Triceps brachii
‖
Contraction
↓
Prime mover

Triceps brachii
‖
Relaxation
↓
Antagonist

The biceps brachii is a primary mover in elbow flexion and the triceps brachii is an antagonist located on the opposite side of the humerus. The prime mover contracts and the antagonist extends to enable smooth joint flexion. In elbow extension, this relationship is reversed so the triceps brachii becomes the primary mover while the biceps brachii becomes the antagonist.

Extension

● **Figure II–19**   Relationship of a primary mover to antagonist in elbow flexion and extension

The synergists are muscles that work to assist the primary movers and the stabilizers are muscles that improve the efficiency of the primary movers by stabilizing the joint. In elbow flexion, for example, the primary movers (biceps brachii, brachialis, and brachioradialis) all contract, while the triceps brachii, on the opposite side of the humerus, relaxes. Thus the distal ends of the radius and ulna are drawn closer to the humerus and flexion of the elbow is smoothly executed. The pronator teres also participates in elbow flexion as a synergist to the primary movers. The deltoid and trapezius are the stabilizers, which maintain the stability in the shoulder joint during elbow flexion. It might seem as if the muscles around the shoulder would not take part in elbow flexion, but they must also be involved in addition to the primary movers.

4) Muscle Groups Involved in Movement

One muscle by itself cannot produce movement in a joint; two or more muscles are always involved. Figures II–20a to II–20c show the muscle groups that alternately act as the primary movers and antagonists in the movement of major joints.

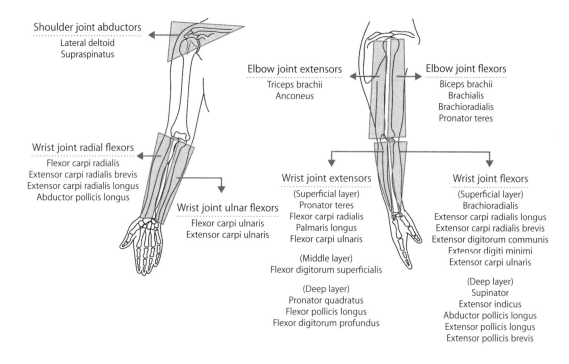

Shoulder joint abductors
Lateral deltoid
Supraspinatus

Elbow joint extensors
Triceps brachii
Anconeus

Elbow joint flexors
Biceps brachii
Brachialis
Brachioradialis
Pronator teres

Wrist joint radial flexors
Flexor carpi radialis
Extensor carpi radialis brevis
Extensor carpi radialis longus
Abductor pollicis longus

Wrist joint ulnar flexors
Flexor carpi ulnaris
Extensor carpi ulnaris

Wrist joint extensors
(Superficial layer)
Pronator teres
Flexor carpi radialis
Palmaris longus
Flexor carpi ulnaris

(Middle layer)
Flexor digitorum superficialis

(Deep layer)
Pronator quadratus
Flexor pollicis longus
Flexor digitorum profundus

Wrist joint flexors
(Superficial layer)
Brachioradialis
Extensor carpi radialis longus
Extensor carpi radialis brevis
Extensor digitorum communis
Extensor digiti minimi
Extensor carpi ulnaris

(Deep layer)
Supinator
Extensor indicus
Abductor pollicis longus
Extensor pollicis longus
Extensor pollicis brevis

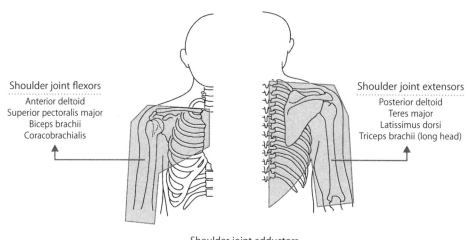

Shoulder joint flexors
Anterior deltoid
Superior pectoralis major
Biceps brachii
Coracobrachialis

Shoulder joint extensors
Posterior deltoid
Teres major
Latissimus dorsi
Triceps brachii (long head)

Shoulder joint adductors
The extensors and flexors of the
shoulder joint work together in
adduction of the arm.

● **Figure II–20a**   Muscle groups involved in movement of shoulders, elbows, and wrists

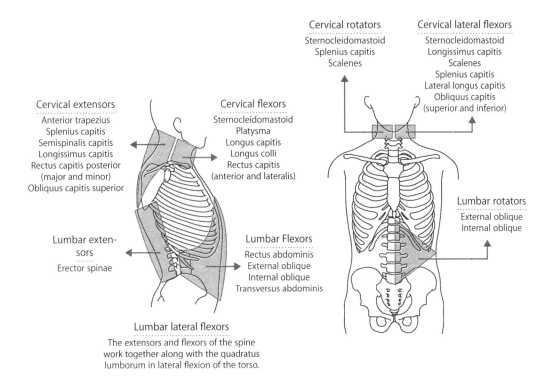

Cervical rotators
Sternocleidomastoid
Splenius capitis
Scalenes

Cervical lateral flexors
Sternocleidomastoid
Longissimus capitis
Scalenes
Splenius capitis
Lateral longus capitis
Obliquus capitis
(superior and inferior)

Cervical extensors
Anterior trapezius
Splenius capitis
Semispinalis capitis
Longissimus capitis
Rectus capitis posterior
(major and minor)
Obliquus capitis superior

Cervical flexors
Sternocleidomastoid
Platysma
Longus capitis
Longus colli
Rectus capitis
(anterior and lateralis)

Lumbar rotators
External oblique
Internal oblique

Lumbar exten-
sors
Erector spinae

Lumbar Flexors
Rectus abdominis
External oblique
Internal oblique
Transversus abdominis

Lumbar lateral flexors
The extensors and flexors of the spine
work together along with the quadratus
lumborum in lateral flexion of the torso.

● **Figure II–20b**   Muscle groups involved in movement of neck and spine

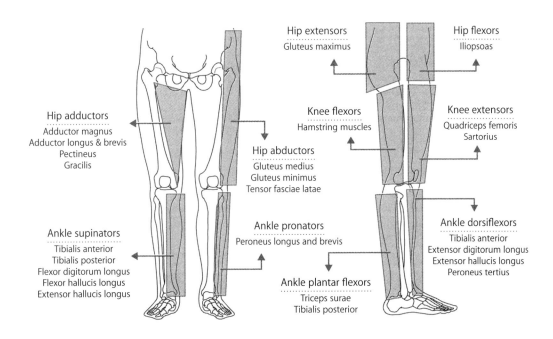

Hip extensors
Gluteus maximus

Hip flexors
Iliopsoas

Hip adductors
Adductor magnus
Adductor longus & brevis
Pectineus
Gracilis

Knee flexors
Hamstring muscles

Knee extensors
Quadriceps femoris
Sartorius

Hip abductors
Gluteus medius
Gluteus minimus
Tensor fasciae latae

Ankle supinators
Tibialis anterior
Tibialis posterior
Flexor digitorum longus
Flexor hallucis longus
Extensor hallucis longus

Ankle pronators
Peroneus longus and brevis

Ankle dorsiflexors
Tibialis anterior
Extensor digitorum longus
Extensor hallucis longus
Peroneus tertius

Ankle plantar flexors
Triceps surae
Tibialis posterior

● **Figure II–20c**   Muscle groups involved in movement of hips, knees, and ankles

B. Extension and Contraction of Muscles with Meridian Test Movements

The muscles on opposite sides of a bone work in a coordinated way, alternately contracting or extending depending on the situation to enable smooth movement in the joint. The muscles on one side contract while those on the other side relax and extend. Each movement of the M-Test stretches certain muscles so that those areas with resistance or impediments to stretching can be located. Both the skin and muscles are involved when there are impediments to stretching, but the muscles by far play the largest part. I will explain which muscles contract and which muscles stretch with each movement of the M-Test (see also the Meridian Test Findings Chart in the Appendix, p. 204.)

1) MUSCLES INVOLVED IN THE MERIDIAN TEST: NECK (FIG. II–21)

a. Anterior aspect

As shown in illustration (1), when the neck is extended, the muscles on the anterior aspect of the neck are stretched. This includes the sternocleidomastoid (SCM) and the platysma, which are located near the surface, and the longus capitis, longus colli, rectus capitis anterior, and rectus capitis lateralis, which are located deeper. These muscles are located on both sides (bilateral) and they are stretched on both sides with neck extension. The oblique extension of the neck, as shown in illustration ②, is a combination of two types of movement: rotation and extension of the neck. The SCM, splenius capitis, and scalenes on the opposite side are stretched in the rotation movement. The SCM, platysma, longus capitis, longus colli, rectus capitis anterior, and rectus capitis lateralis are stretched in the extension movement. As for the SCM, which is involved in both movements, that on the left side is stretched with right oblique rotation, and that on the right side is stretched with left oblique rotation. In the neck rotation movement, shown in illustration ③, the SCM, splenius capitis, and scalenes on the left side are stretched in rotation to the right, and the same muscles on the right side are stretched in rotation to the left.

b. Posterior aspect

As shown in illustration ④, when the neck is flexed, the muscles on the posterior aspect of the neck are stretched. This includes the superior fibers of the trapezius on the surface, the splenius capitis, semispinalis capitis, and longissimus capitis at a medium depth, and the major and minor posterior rectus capitis and superior fibers of the oblique capitis, which are located deeper. These muscles are located

II

A. Anterior Aspect

Meridians
Lung, Large Intestine, Conception

① Extension

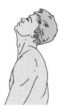

Extended Muscles	Contracted Muscles
Sternocleidomastoid	Superior trapezius
Platysma	Splenius capitis
Longus capitis	Semispinalis capitis
Longus colli	Longissimus capitis
Rectus capitis lateralis and anterior	Rectus capitis posterior major and minor
	Obliquus capitis superior

② Oblique Extension

Extended Muscles	Contracted Muscles
Sternocleidomastoid	Neck extension muscles
Platysma	Neck rotation muscles
Longus capitis	
Longus colli	
Rectus capitis lateralis and anterior	
Splenius capitis	
Scalenes	

③ Rotation

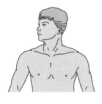

Extended Muscles	Contracted Muscles
Sternocleidomastoid	Same muscles on other side
Splenius capitis	
Scalenes	

B. Posterior Aspect

Meridians
Heart, Small Intestine, Governing

④ Flexion

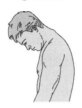

Extended Muscles	Contracted Muscles
Trapezius superior	Sternocleidomastoid
Splenius capitis	Platysma
Semispinalis capitis	Longus capitis
Longissimus capitis	Longus colli
Rectus capitis posterior major and minor	Rectus capitis lateralis and anterior
Obliquus capitis superior	

⑤ Oblique Flexion

Extended Muscles	Contracted Muscles
Trapezius superior	Neck Extension Muscles
Splenius capitis	Neck Rotation Muscles
Semispinalis capitis	
Longissimus capitis	
Rectus capitis posterior major and minor	
Obliquus capitis superior	
Sternocleidomastoid	
Scalenes	

C. Lateral Aspect

Meridians
Pericardium, Triple Burner, Girdle

⑥ Lateral Flexion

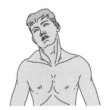

Extended Muscles	Contracted Muscles
Sternocleidomastoid (unilateral)	Same muscles on other side
Longissimus capitis (unilateral)	
Scalenes (unilateral)	
Splenius capitis (unilateral)	
Rectus capitis lateralis (unilateral)	
Obliquus capitis superior and inferior	

Note: Figs II–21 through II–27 are taken from *The Meridian Test*, by Mukaino Yoshito et al, Ishiyaku Shuppan, Tokyo, 1999. Please refer to the Meridian Test Findings Chart in the Appendix, p. 204.

● **Figure II–21** Muscle actions with M-Test: NECK

on both sides (bilateral) and are stretched on both sides with neck flexion. The oblique flexion of the neck, as shown in illustration ⑤, is a combination of two types of movement: rotation and flexion of the neck. The SCM, splenius capitis, and scalenes on the opposite side are stretched in rotation. In flexion, the superior fibers of the trapezius (superficial) are stretched along with the splenius capitis, semispinalis capitis, and longissimus capitis (medium), as well as the major and minor posterior rectus capitis and superior fibers of the oblique capitis (deep).

c. Lateral aspect

As shown in illustration ⑥, when the neck is flexed laterally, the same muscles located on either side of the neck, including the SCM, scalenes, longissimus capitis, splenius capitis, rectus capitis lateralis, and major and minor posterior rectus capitis, are involved. When the neck is flexed to the right, the muscles on the right side contract and the same muscles on the left side are stretched.

2) Muscles Involved in the Meridian Test: Torso (fig. ii–22)

a. Anterior aspect

As shown in illustration ①, the muscles in the torso that are stretched during posterior flexion are the abdominal muscles, including the rectus abdominis, external oblique, and internal oblique, as well as the transversus abdominis, which is located deeper. As is obvious from the illustration, however, along with the muscles in the torso, those on the anterior aspect of the thigh and the neck are also stretched when the body is bent backward. Therefore, when this M-Test for assessing the lumbar region with a back bend is performed, the hip flexors, including the iliopsoas, rectus femoris, and sartorius, are also stretched, along with the neck flexors including the SCM, platysma, longus capitis, longus colli, anterior rectus capitis, and lateral rectus capitis.

b. Posterior aspect

In a similar way, as shown in illustration ②, the muscles stretched during anterior flexion of the torso are not only those of the torso, but also include those in the gluteal region and the posterior thighs, as well as the calves. Therefore, in the forward bending movement of the torso, not only the erector spinae muscles of the back, but the hip extensors, including the gluteus maximus, biceps femoris, semimembranosus, and semitendinosus, are also stretched, along with the ankle flexor, triceps surae.

A. Anterior Aspect	**B. Posterior Aspect**	**C. Lateral Aspect**
Meridians	Meridians	Meridians
Spleen, Stomach, Conception	Kidney, Bladder, Governing	Liver, Gallbladder, Girdle

① **Extension**	② **Flexion**	③ **Rotation**

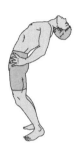
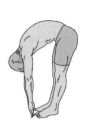
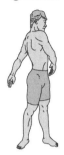

Extended Muscles	Contracted Muscles
Rectus abdominis	Erector spinae
External oblique	
Internal oblique	
Transversus abdominis	

Extended Muscles	Contracted Muscles
Erector spinae	Rectus abdominis
External oblique	
Internal oblique	
Transversus abdominis	

Extended Muscles	Contracted Muscles
External oblique	Same muscles on other side
Internal oblique	

④ **Lateral Flexion**

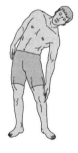

Extended Muscles	Contracted Muscles
Erector spinae	Same muscles on other side
Rectus abdominis	
External oblique	
Internal oblique	
Transversus abdominis	

● **Figure II–22**   Muscle actions with M-Test: TORSO (lumbar area)

c. Lateral aspect

In lateral flexion of the torso, as shown in illustration ④, it is likely that muscles in the lateral aspect of the thigh are stretched along with those in the torso. In other words, when the torso is flexed to the right, the muscles of the torso, including the erector spinae, rectus abdominis, external oblique, internal oblique, and quadratus lumborum, are stretched. Along with this, the hip abductors on the lateral aspect, including the gluteus medius, gluteus minimus, and tensor fasciae latae, are also stretched.

3) Muscles Involved in the Meridian Test: Shoulder (fig. ii–23)

a. Anterior aspect

As shown in illustration ①, the muscles stretched during the extension of the shoulder are the anterior deltoid on the anterior shoulder, the biceps brachii and coracobrachialis of the anterior upper arm, as well as the superior fibers of the pectoralis major. As shown in illustration ②, the same movement with the elbow flexed stretches the same muscles.

When the shoulder joint is rotated medially, the subscapularis, latissimus dorsi, pectoralis major, anterior deltoid, and teres major are contracted, while the posterior deltoid, infraspinatus, and teres minor are stretched. However, when the shoulder is rotated medially after first flexing the elbow and extending the shoulder, as shown in illustration ③, the elbow extensors that are stretched in elbow flexion, as well as the shoulder flexors that are stretched in shoulder extension, are also stretched along with the above-mentioned muscles.

b. Posterior aspect

As shown in illustration ④, the muscles stretched during the flexion of the shoulder are those on the posterior and inferior aspect of the shoulder, including the posterior deltoid, teres major, latissimus dorsi, and the long head of triceps brachii. As shown in illustration ⑤, shoulder flexion with the elbow flexed also stretches the anconeus.

When the shoulder joint is rotated laterally, the posterior deltoid, infraspinatus, and teres minor are contracted, while the subscapularis, latissimus dorsi, pectoralis major, anterior deltoid, and teres major are stretched. However, when the shoulder is rotated laterally after first abducting the shoulder and flexing the elbow, as shown in illustration ⑥, the shoulder adductors and the elbow flexors are also stretched.

c. Lateral aspect

As shown in illustration ⑦, the muscles stretched during horizontal flexion of the shoulder are the muscles on the posterior shoulder region and the lateral aspect of the arm. This includes the posterior deltoid, latissimus dorsi, infraspinatus, teres minor, and the long head of the triceps brachii. When the elbow is flexed during horizontal flexion of the shoulder, as shown in illustration ⑧, a larger area from the elbow to the shoulder is stretched. Thus the anconeus and the short head of triceps brachii are stretched in addition to the above-mentioned muscles.

As shown in illustration ⑨, the muscles stretched during horizontal extension of the shoulder are those on the anterior shoulder

II

A. Anterior Aspect

Meridians
Lung, Large Intestine, Conception

① Extension

Extended Muscles	Contracted Muscles
Anterior deltoid	Posterior deltoid
Superior pectoralis major	Teres major
Biceps brachii	Latissimus dorsi
Coracobrachialis	Triceps brachii (long head)

② Extension with Flexed Elbow

Extended Muscles	Contracted Muscles
Anterior deltoid	Posterior deltoid
Superior pectoralis major	Teres major
Biceps brachii	Latissimus dorsi
Coracobrachialis	Triceps brachii (long head)

③ Medial Rotation with Flexed Elbow

Extended Muscles	Contracted Muscles
Shoulder joint lateral rotators:	Shoulder joint medial rotators:
• Posterior deltoid	• Subscapularis
• Infraspinatus	• Latissimus dorsi
• Teres minor	• Pectoralis major
	• Anterior deltoid
Shoulder joint flexors	• Teres major
Elbow joint extensors	Shoulder joint extensors
	Elbow joint flexors

B. Posterior Aspect

Meridians
Heart, Small Intestine, Governing

④ Flexion

Extended Muscles	Contracted Muscles
Posterior deltoid	Anterior deltoid
Teres major	Superior pectoralis major
Latissimus dorsi	Biceps brachii
Triceps brachii (long head)	Coracobrachialis

⑤ Flexion with Flexed Elbow

Extended Muscles	Contracted Muscles
Posterior deltoid	Anterior deltoid
Teres major	Superior pectoralis major
Latissimus dorsi	Biceps brachii
Triceps brachii	Coracobrachialis
Anconeus	

⑥ Lateral Rotation with Flexed Elbow

Extended Muscles	Contracted Muscles
Shoulder joint medial rotators:	Shoulder joint lateral rotators:
• Subscapularis	• Posterior deltoid
• Latissimus dorsi	• Infraspinatus
• Pectoralis major	• Teres minor
• Anterior deltoid	
• Teres major	
Shoulder joint adductors	Shoulder joint abductors
Elbow joint extensors	Elbow joint flexors

C. Lateral Aspect

Meridians
Pericardium, Triple Burner, Girdle

⑦ Horizontal Flexion

Extended Muscles	Contracted Muscles
Posterior deltoid	Anterior deltoid
Latissimus dorsi	Pectoralis major
Infraspinatu	Coracobrachialis
Teres minor	Subscapularis
Triceps brachii (long head)	Biceps brachii

⑧ Horizontal Flexion with Flexed Elbow

Extended Muscles	Contracted Muscles
Posterior deltoid	Anterior deltoid
Latissimus dorsi	Pectoralis major
Infraspinatus	Coracobrachialis
Teres minor	Subscapularis
Triceps brachii (short head)	Biceps brachii
Anconeus	

⑨ Horizontal Extension

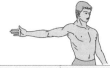

Extended Muscles	Contracted Muscles
Anterior deltoid	Posterior deltoid
Pectoralis major	Latissimus dorsi
Coracobrachialis	Infraspinatus
Subscapularis	Teres minor
Biceps brachii	Triceps brachii (long head)

⑩ Horizontal Extension with Flexed Elbow

Extended Muscles	Contracted Muscles
Anterior deltoid	Posterior deltoid
Pectoralis major	Latissimus dorsi
Coracobrachialis	Infraspinatus
Subscapularis	Teres minor
Biceps brachii	Triceps brachii (long head)

● **Figure II–23**   Muscle actions with M-Test: SHOULDER

region and the anterior aspect of the arm. This includes the anterior deltoid, pectoralis major, coracobrachialis, subscapularis, and biceps brachii. As shown in illustration ⑩, the same muscles are stretched when this movement is performed with the elbow flexed.

4) Muscles Involved in the Meridian Test: Elbow (fig. II–24)

a. Anterior aspect

As shown in illustration ①, the muscles stretched during pronation of the arm are the supinator at the deep level and the biceps brachii on the anterior arm. The muscles of the forearm that originate in the lateral epicondyle of the humerus and insert into the lateral surface of the radius, including the extensor carpi radialis longus and brevis, are also stretched.

b. Posterior aspect

As shown in illustration ②, the muscles stretched during supination of the arm are the pronator teres and pronator quadratus at the deep level. Other muscles stretched in this movement include the flexor carpi ulnaris and flexor digitorum superficialis, which originate on the ulnar aspect of the medial epicondyle of the humerus and insert into the lateral surface of the ulna, as well as the extensor carpi ulnaris and extensor digitorum communis, and extensor digiti minimi, which originate on the lateral epicondyle of the humerus and insert into the lateral surface of the ulna.

c. Lateral aspect

As shown in illustration ③, the muscles stretched during elbow flexion are those on the posterior aspect of the arm such as the triceps brachii and anconeus. These primary movers in elbow flexion originate on the epicondyle of the humerus, pass over the elbow joint, and insert into bones of the forearm. Also stretched in this movement are muscles in the posterior forearm, including the extensor carpi ulnaris, extensor carpi radialis longus and brevis, extensor digitorum, as well as extensor minimi.

As shown in illustration ④, the muscles stretched during extension of the elbow are those on the anterior arm including the biceps brachii, brachialis, brachioradialis, and pronator teres. Since these muscles originate in the upper arm and cross over the elbow joint, the anterior forearm muscles, including the flexor carpi radialis, palmaris longus, flexor carpi ulnaris, and flexor digitorum superficialis, are also slightly stretched.

A. Anterior Aspect	B. Posterior Aspect	C. Lateral Aspect

A. Anterior Aspect

Meridians
Lung, Large Intestine, Conception

① **Pronation**

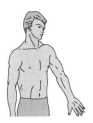

Extended Muscles	Contracted Muscles
Supinator	Pronator
Biceps brachii	Pronator quadratus
Extensor carpi radialis longus/brevis	

B. Posterior Aspect

Meridians
Heart, Small Intestine, Governing

② **Supination**

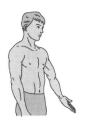

Extended Muscles	Contracted Muscles
Pronator	Supinator
Pronator quadratus	Biceps brachii
Flexor carpi ulnaris	
Flexor digitorum superficialis	
Extensor carpi ulnaris	
Extensor digitorum	
Extensor digiti minimi	

C. Lateral Aspect

Meridians
Pericardium, Triple Burner, Girdle

③ **Flexion**

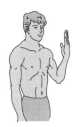

Extended Muscles	Contracted Muscles
Triceps Brachii	Biceps brachii
Anconeus	Brachialis
Extensor carpi ulnaris	Brachioradialis
Extensor carpi radialis longus/brevis	Pronator teres
Extensor digitorum	Flexor carpi radialis
Extensor digiti minimi	Flexor digitorum superficialis

④ **Extension**

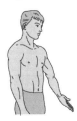

Extended Muscles	Contracted Muscles
Biceps brachii	Triceps Brachii
Brachialis	Anconeus
Brachioradialis	Extensor carpi ulnaris
Pronator teres	Extensor carpi radialis longus/brevis
Flexor carpi radialis	Extensor digitorum
Flexor digitorum superficialis	Extensor digiti minimi

● **Figure II–24** Muscle actions with M-Test: ELBOW

5) Muscles Involved in the Meridian Test: Wrist (Fig. ii–25)

a. Anterior aspect:

As shown in illustration ①, the muscles stretched with adduction (ulnar flexion) of the wrist are those on the radial aspect, including the flexor carpi radialis, extensor carpi radialis longus and brevis, and abductor pollicis longus.

A. Anterior Aspect

Meridians

Lung, Large Intestine, Conception

① **Adduction (ulnar flexion)**

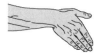

Extended Muscles	Contracted Muscles
Flexor carpi radialis	Flexor carpi ulnaris
Extensor carpi radialis brevis	Extensor carpi ulnaris
Extensor carpi radialis longus	
Abductor pollicis longus	

B. Posterior Aspect

Meridians

Heart, Small Intestine, Governing

② **Abduction (radial flexion)**

Extended Muscles	Contracted Muscles
Flexor carpi ulnaris	Flexor carpi radialis
Extensor carpi ulnaris	Extensor carpi radialis brevis
	Extensor carpi radialis longus
	Abductor pollicis longus

C. Lateral Aspect

Meridians

Pericardium, Triple Burner, Girdle

③ **Flexion**

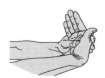

Extended Muscles	Contracted Muscles
Surface Layer:	**Surface Layer:**
Brachioradialis	Pronator teres
Extensor carpi radialis longus	Flexor carpi radialis
Extensor carpi radialis brevis	Palmaris longus
Extensor digitorum	Flexor carpi ulnaris
Extensor digiti minimi	Flexor digitorum superficialis
Middle Layer:	
Extensor carpi ulnaris	
Deep Layer:	**Deep Layer:**
Pronator teres	Pronator quadratus
Extensor indicus	Flexor pollicis longus
Abductor pollicis longus	Flexor digitorum profundus
Extensor digitorum pollicis longus	
Extensor digitorum pollicis brevis	

④ **Extension**

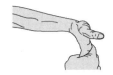

Extended Muscles	Contracted Muscles
Surface Layer:	**Surface Layer:**
Pronator teres	Brachioradialis
Flexor carpi radialis	Extensor carpi radialis longus
Palmaris longus	Extensor carpi radialis brevis
Flexor carpi ulnaris	Extensor digitorum
Middle Layer:	Extensor digiti minimi
Flexor digitorum superficialis	Extensor carpi ulnaris
Deep Layer:	**Deep Layer:**
Pronator quadratus	Pronator teres
Flexor pollicis longus	Extensor indicus
Flexor digitorum profundus	Abductor pollicis longus
	Extensor digitorum pollicis longus
	Extensor digitorum pollicis brevis

● **Figure II–25**   Muscle actions with M-Test: WRIST

b. Posterior aspect

As shown in illustration ②, the muscles stretched with abduction (or radial flexion) of the wrist are those on the ulnar aspect, including the flexor carpi ulnaris and extensor carpi ulnaris.

c. Lateral aspect

Since there are many small muscles in the forearm, I have classified these muscles into those in the superface, middle, and deep layers (Fig. II–16). As shown in illustration ③, the muscles stretched by wrist flexion are the wrist extensors, including the extensor carpi radialis and extensor carpi ulnaris, which originate in the lateral aspect of the forearm and insert into the dorsal aspect of the hand. Also, as shown in illustration ④, the muscles stretched by wrist extension are the wrist flexors, including the flexor carpi radialis and flexor carpi ulnaris, which originate in the medial aspect of the forearm and insert into the palm of the hand.

6) MUSCLES INVOLVED IN THE MERIDIAN TEST: HIP AND KNEE (FIG. II–26)

a. Anterior aspect

As shown in illustration ①, the muscle stretched with hip extension is the iliopsoas on the anterior aspect of the hip joint. At the same time, the rectus femoris, a knee extensor among the quadriceps femoris, is also stretched. The rectus femoris differs from the other three muscles of the quadriceps femoris (vastus lateralis, vastus medialis, and vastus intermedius) in that it originates at the anterior inferior iliac spine. It inserts on the tibia to straddle both the hip joint and the knee joint. This makes the rectus femoris a 'two-joint muscle' that participates in two movements (hip flexion and knee extension). As shown in illustration ②, with knee flexion the muscles of the anterior aspect of the thigh are stretched.

b. Posterior aspect

As shown in illustration ③, mainly the posterior aspect of the thigh is stretched with hip flexion. When the hip is flexed with the ankle in dorsiflexion, in addition to the posterior aspect of the thigh, the posterior aspect of the lower leg and the triceps surae are also stretched. When hip flexion is further increased with simultaneous knee flexion, as shown in illustration ④, the anterior knee and gluteal region are stretched more strongly. Among the muscles of the posterior thigh, the biceps femoris consists of a long and short head. The long head, which originates on the ischial tuberosity, crosses over the two joints of the hip and knee to insert on the head of the fibula. The short head,

A. Anterior Aspect

Meridians
Spleen, Stomach, Conception

① Hip Extension

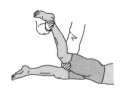

Extended Muscles	Contracted Muscles
Iliopsoas:	Gluteus maximus
• Psoas major	Biceps femoris (long head)
• Iliacus	Semitendinosus
Rectus femoris	Semimembranosus
Sartorius	

② Knee Flexion

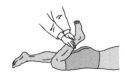

Extended Muscles	Contracted Muscles
Quadriceps femoris:	**Hamstrings:**
• Rectus femoris	• Biceps femoris
• Vastus lateralis	• Semitendinosus
• Vastus medialis	• Semimembranosus
• Vastus intermedius	
Sartorius	

B. Posterior Aspect

Meridians
Kidney, Bladder, Governing

③ Flexion

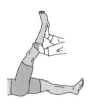

Extended Muscles	Contracted Muscles
Gluteus maximus	**Iliopsoas:**
Biceps femoris	• Psoas major
Semitendinosus	• Iliacus
Semimembranosus	Rectus femoris
	Sartorius

④ Hip Flexion with Knee Flexion

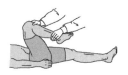

Extended Muscles	Contracted Muscles
Gluteus maximus	**Iliopsoas:**
Biceps femoris (long head)	• Psoas major
Semitendinosus	• Iliacus
Semimembranosus	Rectus femoris
	Sartorius

C. Lateral Aspect

Meridians
Liver, Gallbladder, Girdle

⑤ Abduction

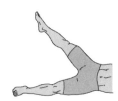

Extended Muscles	Contracted Muscles
Gracilis	Gluteus medius
Adductor magnus	Gluteus minimus
Adductor longus	Tensor fasciae latae
Adductor brevis	
Pectineus	

⑥ Adduction

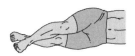

Extended Muscles	Contracted Muscles
Gluteus medius	Gracilis
Gluteus minimus	Adductor magnus
Tensor fasciae latae	Adductor longus
	Adductor brevis
	Pectineus

⑦ Hip External Rotation (Patrick test)

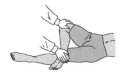

Extended Muscles	Contracted Muscles
Hip joint adductors:	Hip joint flexors
• Gracilis	Hip joint lateral rotators
• Adductor magnus	Hip joint abductors
• Adductor longus	
• Adductor brevis	
• Pectineus	
Hip joint medial rotators:	
• Anterior gluteus medius	
• Gluteus minimus	
• Tensor fasciae latae	
• Semitendinosus	
• Semimembranosus	

● **Figure II–26**   Muscle actions with M-Test: HIP AND KNEE

which originates on the lateral aspect of the femur, crosses over the knee joint and also inserts on the head of the fibula. Because of this, both heads of the biceps femoris are stretched when the hip joint is flexed with the knee extended, but only the long head of biceps femoris is stretched when the hip joint is flexed with the knee flexed.

c. Lateral aspect

As shown in illustration ⑤, the medial aspect of the thigh is stretched with hip abduction. Conversely, in hip adduction, the lateral aspect of the thigh is stretched, as shown in illustration ⑥. The Fabre Patrick test, shown in illustration ⑦, consists of three motions: flexion, abduction, and external rotation of the hip. This movement therefore stretches the muscles that are the antagonists in the above movements (hip extensors, adductors, and medial rotators). The hip adductors are the gracilis, adductor magnus, adductor longus and brevis, and pectineus. The medial rotators of the hip are the anterior fibers of the gluteus medius, the gluteus minimus, tensor fasciae latae, semimembranosus, and semitendinosus. Even though the anterior fibers of the gluteus medius, the gluteus minimus, and tensor fasciae latae are primarily hip abductors, they are also involved in hip adduction. In this M-Test movement (as in the Fabre Patrick test), after placing the leg into the position of hip flexion, abduction, and adduction, the knee is pressed downward to further extend the hip joint. This relaxes the hip extensors, including the gluteus maximus and the long head of biceps femoris, so they are not stretched.

7) Muscles Involved in the Meridian Test: Ankle (fig. ii–27)

a. Anterior aspect

As shown in illustration ①, plantar flexion of the foot mainly stretches the tibialis anterior on the anterior aspect of lower leg. At the same time, the extensor digitorum longus, extensor hallucis longus, and fibularis tertius are also stretched.

b. Posterior aspect

As shown in illustration ②, the muscles stretched in dorsiflexion of the foot are mainly the gastrocnemius and soleus of the triceps surae. The other muscles stretched by this movement include the tibialis posterior, flexor hallucis longus, and flexor digitorum longus (all inferior and posterior to the medial malleolus) as well as the fibularis longus and brevis (both inferior and posterior to the lateral malleolus). The plantaris is a short muscle deep inside the sole, but this dorsiflexion movement also stretches it.

A. Anterior Aspect	B. Posterior Aspect	C. Lateral Aspect

Meridians	Meridians	Meridians
Spleen, Stomach, Conception	Kidney, Bladder, Governing	Liver, Gallbladder, Girdle

① **Plantar Flexion**	② **Dorsiflexion**	③ **Pronation (eversion)**

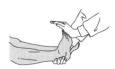
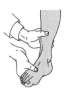

Extended Muscles	Contracted Muscles
Tibialis anterior	Triceps surae:
Extensor digitorum longus	• Gastrocnemius
Extensor hallucis longus	• Soleus
Peroneus tertius	Tibialis posterior
	Flexor digitorum longus
	Flexor hallucis longus
	Peroneus longus
	Peroneus brevis
	Plantaris

Extended Muscles	Contracted Muscles
Tibialis anterior	Peroneus longus
Tibialis posterior	Peroneus brevis
Flexor digitorum longus	Extensor digitorum longus
Flexor hallucis longus	Peroneus tertius
Extensor hallucis longus	

Extended Muscles	Contracted Muscles
Triceps surae:	Tibialis anterior
• Gastrocnemius	Extensor digitorum longus
• Soleus	Extensor hallucis longus
Tibialis posterior	Peroneus tertius
Flexor digitorum longus	
Flexor hallucis longus	
Peroneus longus	
Peroneus brevis	
Plantaris	

④ **Supination (inversion)**

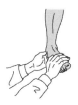

Extended Muscles	Contracted Muscles
Peroneus longus	Tibialis anterior
Peroneus brevis	Tibialis posterior
Extensor digitorum longus	Flexor digitorum longus
Peroneus tertius	Flexor hallucis longus
	Extensor hallucis longus

● **Figure II–27**   Muscle actions with M-Test: ANKLE

c. Lateral aspect

As shown in illustration ③, the muscles stretched in pronation of the foot are the tibialis posterior, flexor digitorum longus, and flexor hallucis longus (all going from the posterior calf to below the medial malleolus) as well as the tibialis anterior and extensor hallucis longus.

As shown in illustration ④, the muscles stretched in supination of the foot are the fibularis longus and brevis (both going inferior and posterior to the lateral malleolus) as well as the extensor digitorum longus and fibularis tertius.

☕ Coffee Break

My Favorite Acupuncture Points

Honda Tatsuro, Acupuncturist at the Wakayama Health Center

Among all the treatments I have done on athletes, low back pain is one of the most common complaints I treat. And if I were asked to list my favorite acupuncture points, it would be the points that are effective for low back pain. Regardless of the type of low back pain, the meridians to be treated are determined by the results of the M-Test. So I don't use these points for all cases of low back pain, but even so, they are my favorite points that I end up using frequently because they are so effective. These points are as follows (see Fig. II–28):

● GALLBLADDER MERIDIAN OF THE LEG

1. **GB-26** *(Daimai)*: Below the anterior tip of the eleventh rib, at the level of the umbilicus.

2. **GB-30** *(Huantiao)*: At the lateral end of the hip joint crease when the hip is fully flexed in side-lying position; in the depression anterior to the greater trochanter.

3. **GB-31** *(Fengshi)*: On the lateral aspect of the thigh, halfway between the greater trochanter and the knee. At the level of the tip of the middle finger when standing straight with the arms at the side.

● LIVER MERIDIAN OF THE LEG

4. **LR-9** *(Yinbao)*: On the medial thigh, one-third the distance from the medial epicondyle of the femur up to the pubic symphysis; between the sartorius and the gracilis muscles.

● SPLEEN MERIDIAN OF THE LEG

5. **SP-6** *(Sanyinjiao)*: On the medial thigh one-fifth the distance from the medial malleolus up to the knee joint; on the posterior border of the tibia.

I use points (1) through (4) primarily for low back pain caused by fatigue in the lateral aspect of the legs. Be that as it may, in addition to treating the lateral aspect, I have used these points to good effect for strains in the anterior and posterior aspects. I wondered why this was, and I gave it some thought. I realized that perhaps the lateral aspect

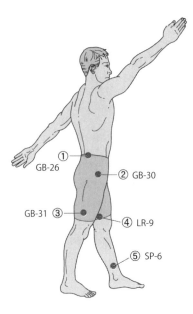

● **Figure II–28**   My favorite acupuncture points

(including the medial and lateral sides) lies in the middle between the anterior and posterior aspects and thus is involved to some extent in assisting movements in the anterior and posterior aspects. Therefore, in cases where good results aren't forthcoming with treatment for the anterior and posterior aspects, treating points (1) through (4) on the lower limb helps improve motion and yields better results.

In the M-Test method, SP-6 is normally a point used when restrictions have been found in the anterior aspect. Perhaps because it is traditionally known as the point where the three yin meridians of the leg cross, in many cases it is effective for restrictions on the medial side. Fatigue in the lower limbs can probably be eliminated more completely if these points are thoroughly massaged on the athlete. In any case, these five points have become indispensable points that I rely on in critical situations. ●

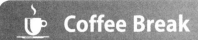

Coffee Break

My Most Memorable Case

Honda Tatsuro, Acupuncturist at the Wakayama Health Center

Among the many treatments I have given to athletes, there is one that remains especially vivid in my memory. It was a series of treatments

II

given to a male table tennis player. Someone asked me to see an athlete competing in the National Athletic Meet for a certain prefecture who had terrible back pain and was in danger of missing the meet. His prefecture was aiming for the championship (in table tennis), and this athlete was one of the hopefuls.

I saw this athlete the next day. He walked into my office dragging his feet. I still distinctly recall the scene, and I thought to myself, "I sure have taken on a difficult case." The athlete told me he had to leave for the National Athletic Meet nine days later. Of these nine days, there were five in which our schedules just did not work. So I could treat him only four times. I asked him to be prepared to receive intensive treatments. Actually, I had experience treating athletes intensively (everyday) as a sports trainer, so I was sure I could do this without exacerbating his symptoms.

I questioned this athlete thoroughly and learned that, among other things, he had received a diagnosis of lumbar disk herniation. Next I performed the M-Test, especially focusing on movements of the lower half of the body. Based on the results I identified the area of treatment and applied a combination of techniques that seemed beneficial including acupuncture, massage, and stretching. I was able to confirm the improvement together with the athlete as this series of treatments progressed. By the fourth and final treatment, the pain was down to 20 percent of what it had been when he first came in. I concluded the fourth treatment with words of encouragement: "The pain has decreased this much and the movement in your body has improved greatly, so all you have to do now is give it your best."

I never heard back from the athlete after that so I just thought to myself that either the pain had become worse so that he couldn't take part in the competition, or that the pain had prevented him from performing optimally, and he found it difficult to report back to me. I was very busy after that so I forgot to check up on the performance of that athlete in the National Athletic Meet. But sometime later I had a chance to talk with the person who introduced the athlete to me, so I asked, "How did that guy I treated a while back do in the National Athletic Meet?"

I was told that although he had experienced some pain during the games, he was able to perform well and went on to win the championship. This was great news after I had almost forgotten about it! I was very glad to learn that the athlete recovered from severe low back pain and was able to perform at almost 100 percent. Not only that, but he had won the championship at the National Athletic Meet, and this episode became etched in my memory as a top prize. ●

☕ Coffee Break

Athletes and Acupuncture Treatments

Honda Tatsuro, Acupuncturist at the Wakayama Health Center

This is a story from when I was still an assistant trainer at a university. I was having a conversation with a female Olympic athlete. I casually asked her, "Have you ever had acupuncture?" This athlete responded, "It's never entered my mind to get acupuncture. They stick needles into your muscles, you know!" This response was an unexpected one for me as I was interested in learning acupuncture. Probably she shared her honest feelings about acupuncture with me because I was just an assistant trainer and not an acupuncturist. I may not have got the same answer if I had asked after already being qualified as an acupuncturist. To top athletes, muscles are important things that enable the body to move. She must have thought that something terrible could happen if needles were inserted into her precious muscles.

By way of contrast, another story concerns a male athlete who always seemed to be dissatisfied with the acupuncture treatments I gave him. This man had once been a representative of his sport for Japan, and was well known in his field. He told me, "A long time ago I was injured before an important match and I couldn't heal from it even after making the rounds of medical clinics. I got acupuncture from a certain doctor and I was able to make the match. That doctor used specially ordered thick needles, so my body may not respond unless the needles are long and thick." So, while this athlete believed in the efficacy of acupuncture, he was fixated on strong stimulation.

In this way, attitudes toward acupuncture vary among athletes, just as with the general public. It might be necessary sometimes for those of us who provide acupuncture treatments to be flexible and take into consideration the preferences of the athlete when we decide the mode of acupuncture and overall treatment strategy. It seems that top athletes worry more about the possible damage to their bodies with acupuncture than they do about the pain (needle sensation).

So we should pay attention to the thoughts and feelings of athletes as we give treatments. I pay careful attention to those I treat for the first time so that I don't inadvertently create associations of fear or discomfort about acupuncture. For this reason, in the initial consultation, I always ask about the level of fear of needles, and whether they have previous experience with acupuncture. It is not true that the effect of acupuncture depends on the insertion of long or big needles.

Surprising results can be obtained with short and thin needles. So, for athletes who are reluctant to be treated with long needles, as in my first story, I show them press tacks and intradermal needles, which are extremely short. I think it is important to show them that we can also use needles that never reach the muscles and are completely safe. •

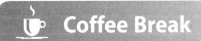

The Seventh Rule of the Meridian Test Must be Followed!

Sawazaki Kenta, Instructor at Fukuoka School for the Blind

Students of the Sports Science Department come for acupuncture treatments at the clinic of the Sports Medicine Department of Fukuoka University, so we see many interesting cases related to movement in sports. One day a 21-year-old female student came in after suffering low back pain for three days. She had a yacht race coming up in two days at the National Athletic Meet. Her pain was at its worst with extension of the trunk.

Since there was pain with extension, I decided there was restriction in the stretching movement of the anterior aspect. To treat the low back pain, I stimulated acupuncture points on the lower half of her body on the Stomach and Spleen meridians, which cover the anterior aspect.

The positive findings in the M-Test for the lower limbs, and my point selection, were as follows: For restriction in extension of both legs, ST-36 and SP-6 (on the lower leg) were treated with press tacks. For restriction in flexion of the right knee, ST-25 (on the abdomen) and ST-34 and SP-10 (just above the knee) were treated with press tacks. The restriction in extension of the legs was reduced, so I had the patient try trunk extension to see if this still caused low back pain. There was not much improvement, however, in the low back pain caused by trunk extension. If the original pain level was a 10, it had only changed to about an 8. After this I did more acupuncture at reactive points on the anterior aspect of the lower body, as well as the area of pain, but this didn't bring much relief either.

I didn't have much knowledge about the sport of yachting, but I thought I might get some ideas for treatment, so I decided to question this patient in detail about the characteristic movements in yachting. In order to raise or hold sails under conditions of strong winds, of course, she had to lean over backward or extend her torso. In addition, I learned that she held the sails up by grasping and pulling on ropes. These strong pulling (extension) movements with her arms placed a lot of stress on her upper body. Based on this information, I performed the M-Test movements for the upper body and found that the low back pain occurred with extension of both the right and left arms. I placed press tacks in LU-1 and LI-11 (points associated with the anterior aspect of the upper body) to treat the restriction in extension of the arms. This brought dramatic improvement and reduced the back pain caused by extension of the torso to about 1 out of 10.

Because this student had presented with low back pain, I had focused on the lower half of her body, but I realized that restrictions in the upper half of the body have a big influence on low back pain as well. Her low back pain had all but disappeared the next day, and this athlete reported to me later that she had done very well and placed second at the National Athletic Meet. This was a case that impressed upon me the need to follow the seventh rule of the M-Test: "Be sure to check all the movements first." •

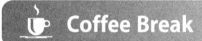

Coffee Break

A Gold Medal from the Meridian Test Method?

Sawazaki Kenta, Instructor at Fukuoka School for the Blind

The Pan-Pacific Swim Meet, in which countries around the Pacific (including the United States) participate, was held in Fukuoka, Japan in the summer of 1997. Among the participating teams, there was one that did not have a sports trainer accompany them, so I was given the opportunity to participate in this meet as the trainer for swimmers of that country. Halfway into the meet, fatigue set in among the swimmers, and I repeatedly encountered situations where no matter how much I massaged the local areas, the tension in the shoulders and the hamstrings could not be relieved. One swimmer could not swim as well as he had intended and therefore had to forfeit the semifinals and the finals in the butterfly. This was actually a sacrifice to save himself for the most important event scheduled for the following day, the 50-meter freestyle.

The swimmer's condition after returning to the hotel was still no better, and the coach was hanging around with a worried expression. After a while, the swimmer, who had refused acupuncture until then, said "I want to try acupuncture." This was back when I had less than a year's experience after obtaining my acupuncture license, so I felt a bit uncertain. Anyway, I went right ahead and performed the M-Test to

II

assess the movements of the whole body and used press tacks for the treatment. Right after this treatment, the tension in his shoulders and hamstrings that formerly would not relax disappeared completely. It seems that his shoulder tension had to do with arm movements, and the tension in his hamstrings was related to ankle movements. This swimmer was very surprised by the effects of the acupuncture treatment, and I was even more surprised than the swimmer. After that I gave a similar treatment to the coach, who had been looking on as if he couldn't quite believe what was happening. Once he had personally experienced the effect of acupuncture through the application of the M-Test, he became convinced and was very happy,

The next morning was the last day of the meet when the 50-meter freestyle races took place. When I went up to our swimmer who was warming up in the sub-pool, even to my inexperienced eyes it was clear that he was swimming freely and smoothly. He welcomed me with a big smile saying, "Thanks to acupuncture my movements are light and free." Our swimmer placed third in the semifinals that morning and was selected to go on to the final race. The anticipated finals took place that afternoon. The race was a dead heat near the end when our swimmer caught up with an American swimmer who was in the lead. Our swimmer won by the narrowest of margins, and not only did he win the gold medal, but he set a new record for himself.

Through this experience at the Pan-Pacific Swim Meet in Fukuoka, I became convinced that acupuncture using the M-Test method could play an important role not only in treating injuries, but also in maximizing conditioning. ●

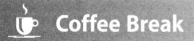

Coffee Break

What I Think is Important in Treatment

Honda Tatsuro, Acupuncturist at the Wakayama Health Center

The thing I emphasize in giving treatments is to place my hands on the patient and touch the restricted area identified by the M-Tests.

I try to think as little as possible as I palpate the restricted area and the associated meridians. I press points successively to assess the condition of the skin and muscles in these areas. This also provides beneficial stimulation, much like massage and shiatsu. I became keenly aware of the importance of touching the patient's body and problem area when I was working with athletes as a trainer. An athletic trainer is like a jack-of-all-trades. The trainer must provide anything the athletes might need including taping, icing, massage, acupuncture, reha-bilitation exercises, and training advice. It is not sufficient to simply give acupuncture and moxibustion treatments. I learned the value of touching the body in this demanding environment.

Many athletes are relieved when the area of pain or fatigue is touched, and some appreciate the treatment more when it is hands-on. Also, for my part, I learned to feel the subtle differences in the texture of the skin and muscles in my fingertips by making a habit of palpating the restricted areas in all the athletes I treat. Often I find indurations or tension in muscles in the areas that are fatigued by repeated movements. And quite often these indurations correspond to the location of acupuncture points. I sometimes think that acu-puncture points were identified in places that are stressed with move-ment or carry a load.

I feel that one of the merits of the M-Test method is that by checking various movements, in addition to the meridians and points, one can easily identify which part of the body needs to be palpated. Of course, massage or stretching can be applied directly to this area as well. I consider assessing the condition of the restricted area by palpa-tion to be as important as inserting the needles into the acupuncture points. •

References

1. Mukaino Yoshito, Gerald Kolblinger, and Chen Yong, *Keiraku Tesuto* (Meridian Test), Ishiyaku Shuppan, 1999.
2. Booher, James M., and Thibodeau, Gary A., *Athletic Injury Assessment*: 3rd ed: Times Mirror/Mosby College, St. Louis, 1989. Japanese translation supervised by Watanabe Yoshihiro, published by Nishimu-ra Shoten, Niigata, Japan, 1993.
3. Floyd, R.T. and Thompson, C.W., *Manual of Structural Kinesiology*. WCB/McGraw-Hill, 13th ed., 1998.
4. Farrar, W.W. and Byrd, S.: *Human Anatomy, Laboratory Manual and Lecture Workbook*, McGraw-Hill Companies, New York, 1997.

SECTION III

**The Practice of
Sports Acupuncture**

1

....

The Practice of the Meridian Test

by Sawazaki Kenta

A. The Meridian Test Protocol (see steps 1, 2 & 3)

THE MERIDIAN TEST ('M-TEST') originally consisted of thirty-one movements, including four movements each for the neck and spine, eight movements for the arm, seven movements for the leg, and four movements each for the hand and foot. These movements or 'tests' are designed to identify restrictions in the anterior, posterior, and lateral (including medial) aspects of the body. (See also the Meridian Test Findings Chart in the appendix.) I have summarized the benefits of the M-Test in Figure III–1, placed the five steps for applying the M-Test in Figure III–2, and listed the seven basic rules of the M-Test in Figure III–3. In this chapter I will introduce the M-Test protocol with the use of illustrations and photos so that it can be applied easily and quickly in the field where athletes need the care. I will also describe the corresponding abnormal areas, meridians, and acupuncture points with the use of illustrations, naming only the primary muscles and essential points.

B. Approaches to Treatment (see steps 4 & 5)

The effect of acupuncture points selected for treatment based on the M-Test is confirmed when symptoms such as pain improve and consequently the associated movement also improves. Thus when a symptom such as pain is associated with a particular movement, finger pressure is applied on the related tender points or key points corresponding to the abnormal area. The best points for treatment

Movements in sports can be assessed.

When movements are assessed using the M-Test, in addition to individual joints involved in sports activities, movements involving multiple joints across the limbs and torso can be analyzed to identify symptoms and imbalances.

The acupuncture points and abnormal areas can be identified.

When movements are assessed using the M-Test, the acupuncture meridians and points of Oriental medicine, and the abnormal areas (muscles, tendons, and ligaments etc.) of Western medicine, can be identified. Thus injury prevention, conditioning, and performance enhancement can be done effectively.

Treatment and prevention can be effected.

When movements are assessed using the M-Test, even if one doesn't have specialized knowledge, the acupuncture points and abnormal areas can be identified based upon the restricted movements. Moreover, abnormal areas can be stretched and massaged, or widely available tapes or plasters can be applied, to treat the problem and prevent injuries.

Self-conditioning can be done on a daily basis.

When movements are assessed using the M-Test, it only takes about ten minutes, so it can be easily done on oneself on a regular basis. Thus it can be applied broadly for self-conditioning on a daily basis.

- **Figure III–1**   What the M-Test can do

1. The M-Test Protocol

STEP ❶ **Perform the M-Test.**

Check for abnormalities in movement with the M-Test Findings Chart (p. 204).

STEP ❷ **Identify abnormal areas or aspects.**

Find the abnormal areas based on abnormal movements.

STEP ❸ **Select the acupuncture points to treat.**

Select the primary points from those in the abnormal area.

2. Approach to Treatment

STEP ❹ **Confirm the effect of the points.**

Check the effect of the points and choose the most effective ones.

STEP ❺ **Treat using the chosen approach.**

Treat the affected area by stimulating points or by other means.

- **Figure III–2**   The five steps of the M-Test

1. Check all of the movements first.

2. Treat the meridian with the greatest restriction first.

3. When the abnormality affects both an arm and a leg, always begin with treatment of the leg.

4. Do not forget to stimulate the central axis.

5. Before treating a point, first check its effect by striking or applying pressure to see if it improves the movement.

6. Stimulation of the local area should be done last.

7. If there is no effect with treatment, refer to an orthopedist or other health professional.

- **Figure II–3**   Seven rules for the M-Test

are those which reduce or eliminate the various symptoms associated with problematic movements. Even if a symptom is alleviated temporarily, there is often a recurrence of restriction in movement. Therefore treatment should aim for long-term results by repeatedly seeking improvement in the symptom and range of motion. Where repeated attempts yield no improvement in subjective symptoms or in the range of motion, however, the patient must be referred to a physician without delay for a thorough examination. (See Fig. III–35, Step ❹, Confirm the Effect of Points.)

1. ACUPUNCTURE AND MOXIBUSTION (FOR ACUPUNCTURISTS AND MEDICAL PROFESSIONALS)

In sports acupuncture, disposable filiform needles or intradermal needles (press tacks) are used (Fig. III–4). The disposable press tacks are very easy to use and can reduce the time it takes to give a treatment, especially in the field. Since the diameter of these needles is 0.1 to 0.2mm and the length is only about 1mm, it practically eliminates potential problems such as damage to nerves, blood vessels, and muscle tissue, as well as infection. Press tacks are therefore highly recommended from the standpoint of safety.

For moxibustion, or the stimulation of acupuncture points with heat, the products readily available in Japan that do not leave a burn on the skin are recommended. These include Sennen Kyu and Kamaya Mini (stick-on moxa cones with adhesive on the bottom; see Fig. III–5). For reasons of safety and expedience, these products are also recommended in the field, or for self-treatment at home.

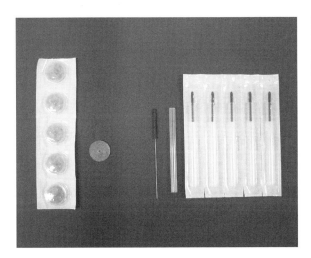

● **Figure III–4**   Intradermal needles (press tacks) and Seirin needles

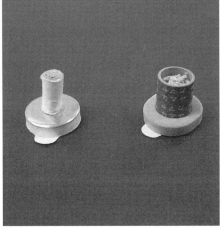

● **Figure III–5**   Varieties of moxibustion with adhesive

2. STRETCHING (FOR THE GENERAL PUBLIC AND SPORTS TRAINERS)

When restrictions in movement and problematic areas are identified by the M-Test, appropriate stretching can be effective for self-conditioning and prevention of injury. Also, applying finger pressure on corresponding points during the stretching is effective for increasing the range of motion. (See Fig. III–36 to 38, Step ❺ Treat Using Chosen Approach — stretching)

3. MASSAGE, TAPING, AND PLASTERS (FOR THE GENERAL PUBLIC, SPORTS TRAINERS, AND MASSAGE THERAPISTS)

Massage is a very effective modality for treating athletes. When giving a treatment, a massage therapist generally palpates all over the body to determine which areas need to be massaged. When the M-Test is performed first to identify the area most in need of treatment, even novices can apply massage quite effectively in the field as well as at home (Fig. III–6, 7 & 8).

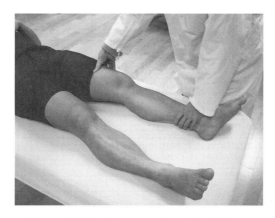

● **Figure III–6**   Massage of anterior thigh

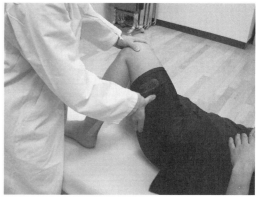

● **Figure III–7**   Massage of lateral thigh

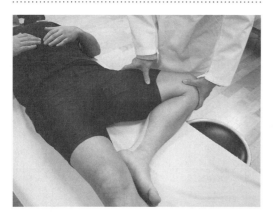

● **Figure III–8**   Massage of medial thigh

Plasters and tape can also be applied to indicated skin surfaces (Fig. III–9 & 10). Kinesio-Tape is a popular Japanese medical product that is applied in sports medicine. If taping causes itching or skin irritation, silk tape can be substituted. Apply the plaster or tape to those places identified as abnormal in Step ❷ of the M-Test. When tape is indicated, pieces 2 to 3cm in width and 10 to 20cm in length are generally sufficient. Since the effects of plasters and tape do not last very long, and can sometimes irritate the skin, it is recommended that they be removed after 24 hours. There are other popular Japanese medical products, such a stick-on magnets and pellets, which also have an effect by putting pressure on the points. There are many ways that such devices can be improvised, such as by cutting off the end of a Q-tip and taping it on a point.

III

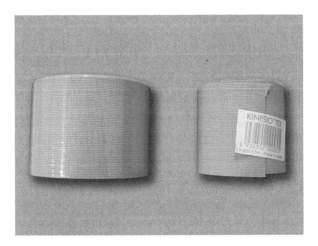

● **Figure III–9**   Kinesio-Tape

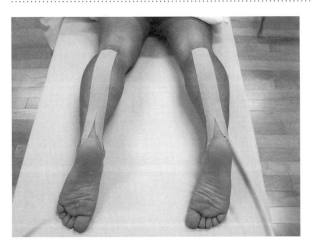

● **Figure III–10**   Kinesio-Tape on posterior calves

STEP **1** **Perform the M-Test**   NECK MOVEMENTS

1. Extension

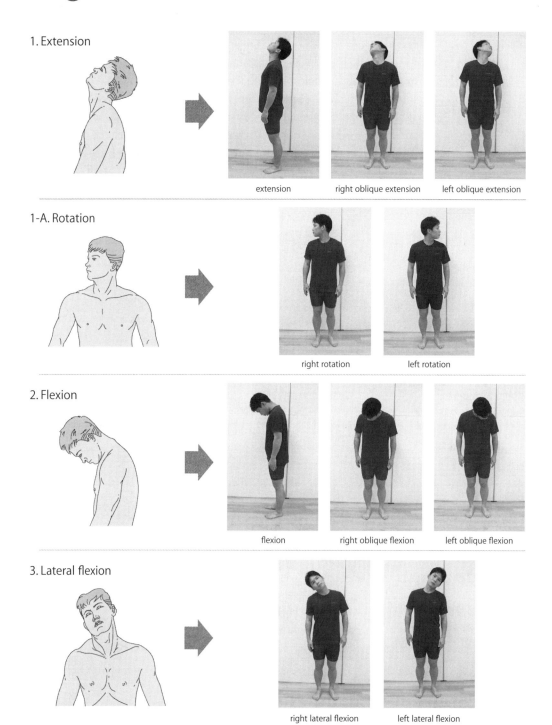

extension   right oblique extension   left oblique extension

1-A. Rotation

right rotation   left rotation

2. Flexion

flexion   right oblique flexion   left oblique flexion

3. Lateral flexion

right lateral flexion   left lateral flexion

● **Figure III–11**

STEP **1** **Perform the M-Test**   ARM MOVEMENTS

III

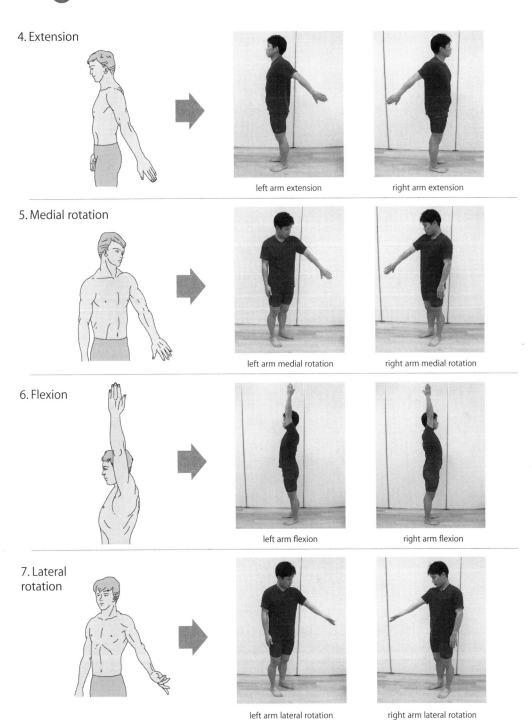

4. Extension

left arm extension   right arm extension

5. Medial rotation

left arm medial rotation   right arm medial rotation

6. Flexion

left arm flexion   right arm flexion

7. Lateral rotation

left arm lateral rotation   right arm lateral rotation

● **Figure III–12**

STEP **1** **Perform the M-Test**   ARM MOVEMENTS

8. Horizontal flexion

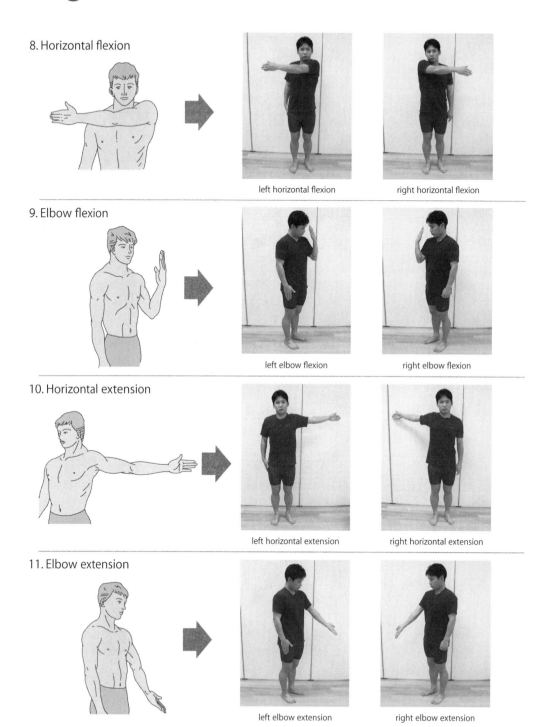

left horizontal flexion

right horizontal flexion

9. Elbow flexion

left elbow flexion

right elbow flexion

10. Horizontal extension

left horizontal extension

right horizontal extension

11. Elbow extension

left elbow extension

right elbow extension

● **Figure III–13**

STEP **1** **Perform the M-Test**   WRIST MOVEMENTS

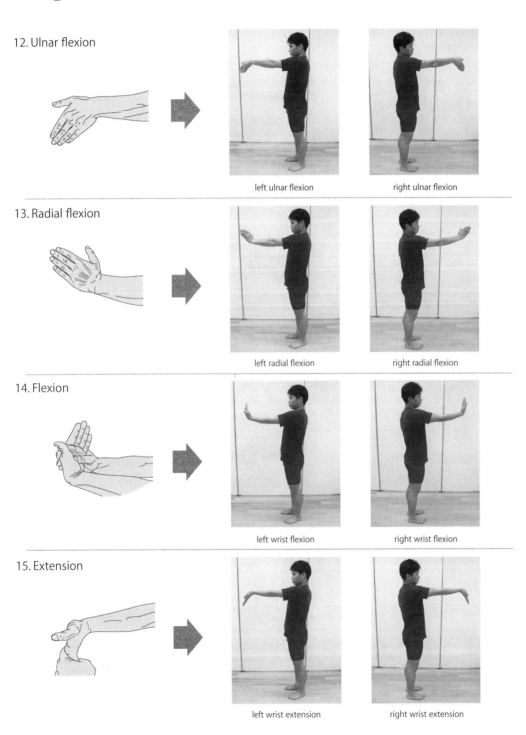

12. Ulnar flexion

left ulnar flexion   right ulnar flexion

13. Radial flexion

left radial flexion   right radial flexion

14. Flexion

left wrist flexion   right wrist flexion

15. Extension

left wrist extension   right wrist extension

● **Figure III–14**

STEP ① **Perform the M-Test**   LEG MOVEMENTS

16. Extension

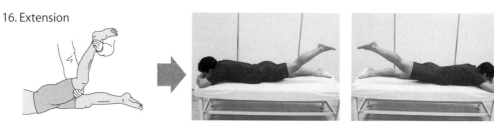

left *leg* extension   right *leg* extension

17. Knee flexion

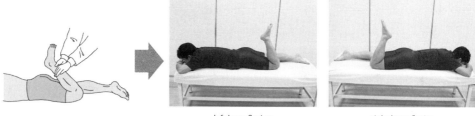

left knee flexion   right knee flexion

18. Flexion

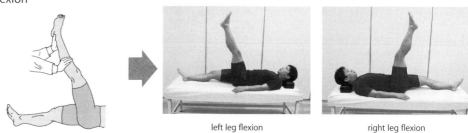

left leg flexion   right leg flexion

19. Hip & knee flexion

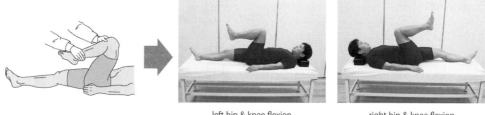

left hip & knee flexion   right hip & knee flexion

● **Figure III–15**

STEP **1** **Perform the M-Test**   LEG MOVEMENTS

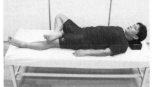

20. Lateral rotation

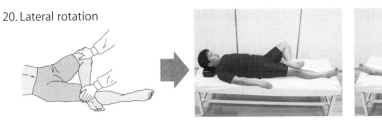

left lateral rotation   right lateral rotation

21. Adduction

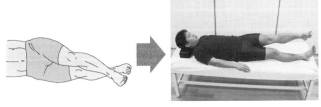
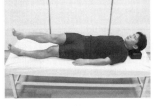

left adduction   right adduction

22. Abduction

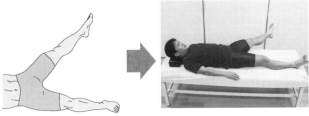

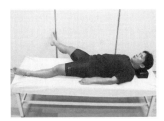

left abduction   right abduction

● **Figure III–16**

STEP **1** **Perform the M-Test**   ANKLE MOVEMENTS

23. Plantar flexion

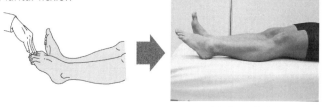

left plantar flexion   right plantar flexion

24. Dorsiflexion

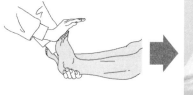
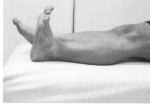
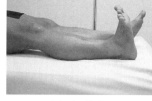

left dorsiflexion   right dorsiflexion

25. Supination

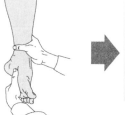
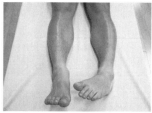
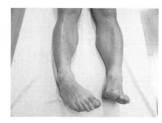

left supination   right supination

26. Pronation

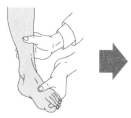
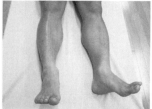
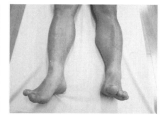

left pronation   right pronation

● **Figure III–17**

STEP **1** **Perform the M-Test**   TORSO MOVEMENTS

27. Extension

28. Flexion

29. Lateral flexion

30. Rotation

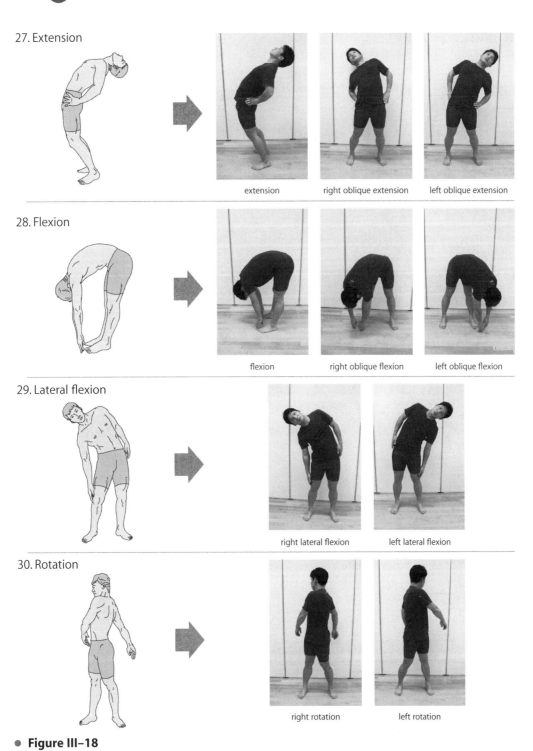

extension   right oblique extension   left oblique extension

flexion   right oblique flexion   left oblique flexion

right lateral flexion   left lateral flexion

right rotation   left rotation

● **Figure III–18**

STEP **2** **Identify the Abnormal Areas (Aspects)**   ANTERIOR UPPER BODY

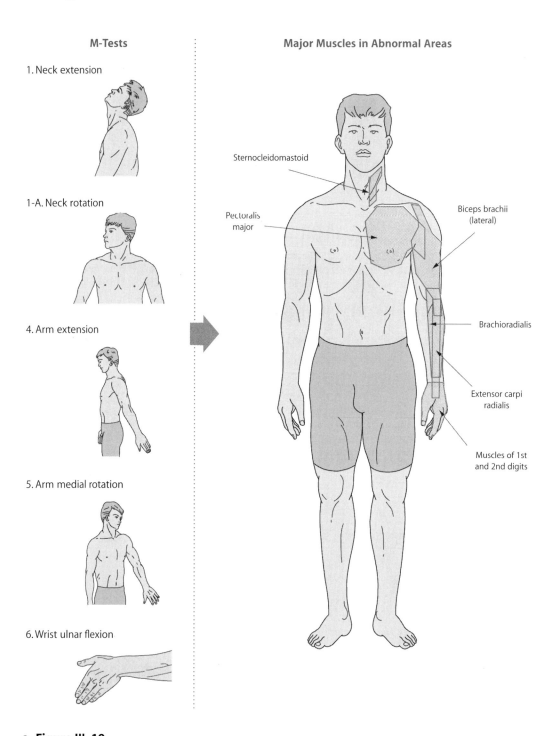

M-Tests	Major Muscles in Abnormal Areas

1. Neck extension

1-A. Neck rotation

4. Arm extension

5. Arm medial rotation

6. Wrist ulnar flexion

Sternocleidomastoid

Pectoralis major

Biceps brachii (lateral)

Brachioradialis

Extensor carpi radialis

Muscles of 1st and 2nd digits

● **Figure III–19**

STEP **2** **Identify Abnormal Areas (Aspects)** POSTERIOR UPPER BODY

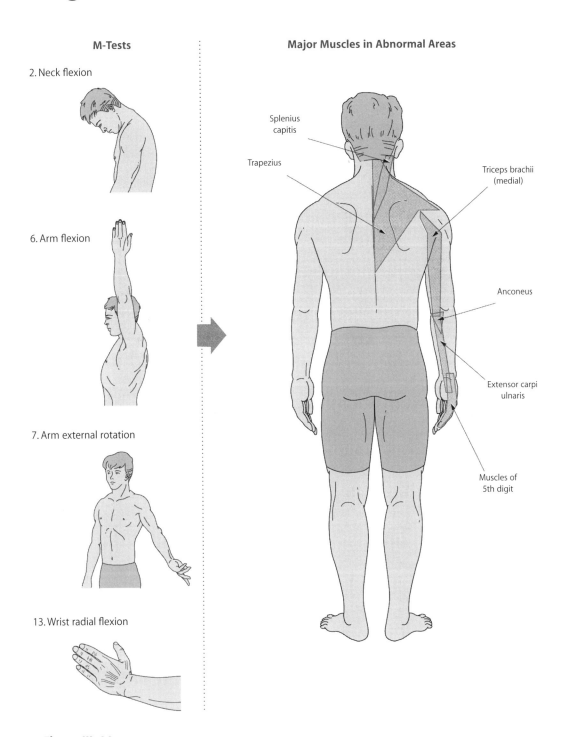

M-Tests

2. Neck flexion

6. Arm flexion

7. Arm external rotation

13. Wrist radial flexion

Major Muscles in Abnormal Areas

Splenius
capitis

Trapezius

Triceps brachii
(medial)

Anconeus

Extensor carpi
ulnaris

Muscles of
5th digit

● **Figure III–20**

STEP **2** **Identify Abnormal Areas (Aspects)** LATERAL UPPER BODY

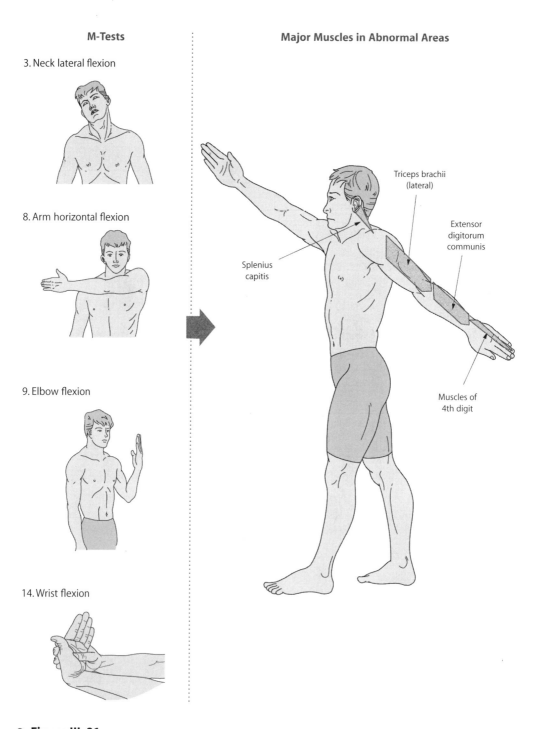

M-Tests

3. Neck lateral flexion

8. Arm horizontal flexion

9. Elbow flexion

14. Wrist flexion

Major Muscles in Abnormal Areas

Splenius capitis

Triceps brachii (lateral)

Extensor digitorum communis

Muscles of 4th digit

● **Figure III–21**

STEP **②** **Identify Abnormal Areas (Aspects)**   MEDIAL UPPER BODY   III

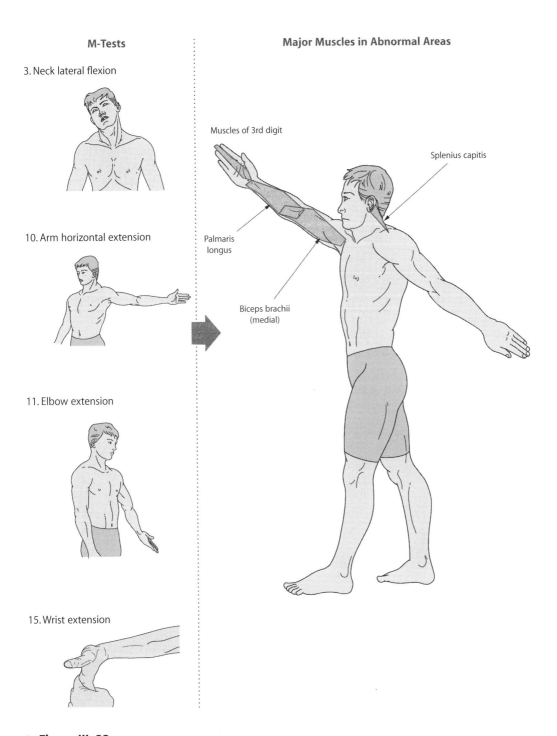

M-Tests

3. Neck lateral flexion

10. Arm horizontal extension

11. Elbow extension

15. Wrist extension

Major Muscles in Abnormal Areas

Muscles of 3rd digit

Splenius capitis

Palmaris longus

Biceps brachii (medial)

● **Figure III–22**

STEP **2** **Identify Abnormal Areas (Aspects)**   ANTERIOR LOWER BODY

M-Tests

16. Hip extension

17. Knee flexion

23. Plantar flexion

27. Torso extension

Major Muscles in Abnormal Areas

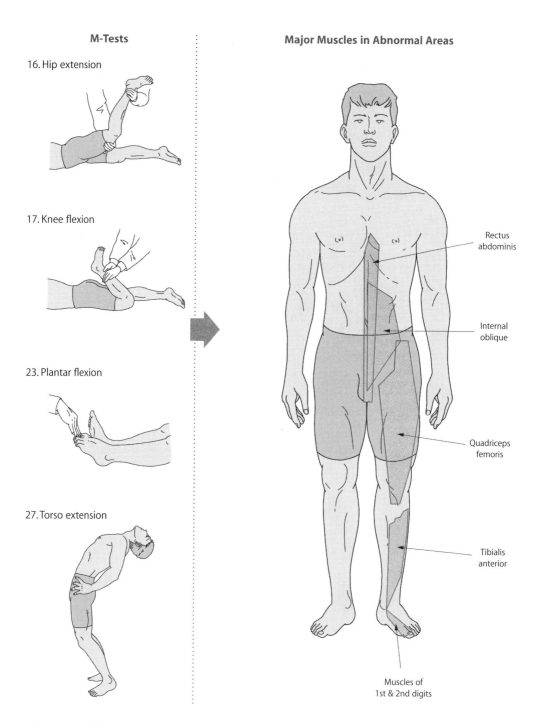

Rectus abdominis

Internal oblique

Quadriceps femoris

Tibialis anterior

Muscles of 1st & 2nd digits

● **Figure III–23**

STEP **②** **Identify Abnormal Areas (Aspects)**   POSTERIOR LOWER BODY   III

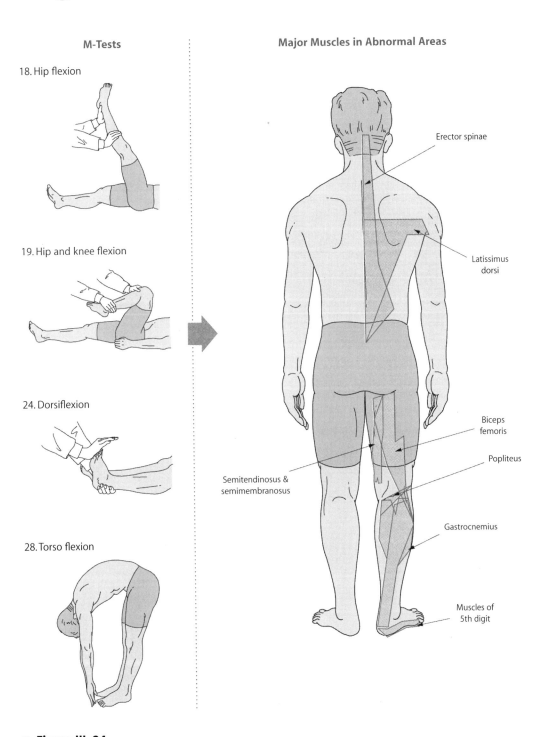

M-Tests

18. Hip flexion

19. Hip and knee flexion

24. Dorsiflexion

28. Torso flexion

Major Muscles in Abnormal Areas

Erector spinae

Latissimus dorsi

Biceps femoris

Popliteus

Semitendinosus & semimembranosus

Gastrocnemius

Muscles of 5th digit

● **Figure III–24**

STEP ❷ **Identify Abnormal Areas (Aspects)**   LATERAL LOWER BODY

M-Tests

20. Hip lateral flexion

22. Hip abduction

25. Ankle supination

29. Torso lateral flexion

30. Torso rotation

Major Muscles in Abnormal Areas

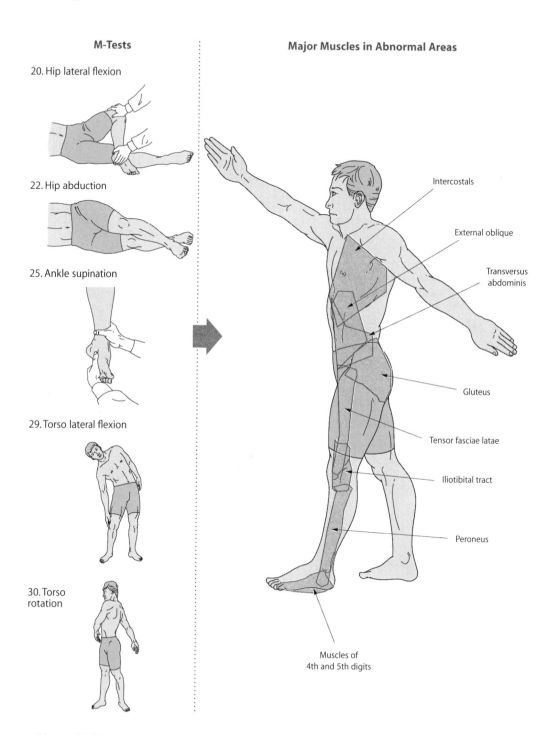

Intercostals

External oblique

Transversus abdominis

Gluteus

Tensor fasciae latae

Iliotibital tract

Peroneus

Muscles of
4th and 5th digits

● **Figure III–25**

STEP ❷ **Identify Abnormal Areas (Aspects)**   MEDIAL LOWER BODY |||

M-Tests   Major Muscles in Abnormal Areas

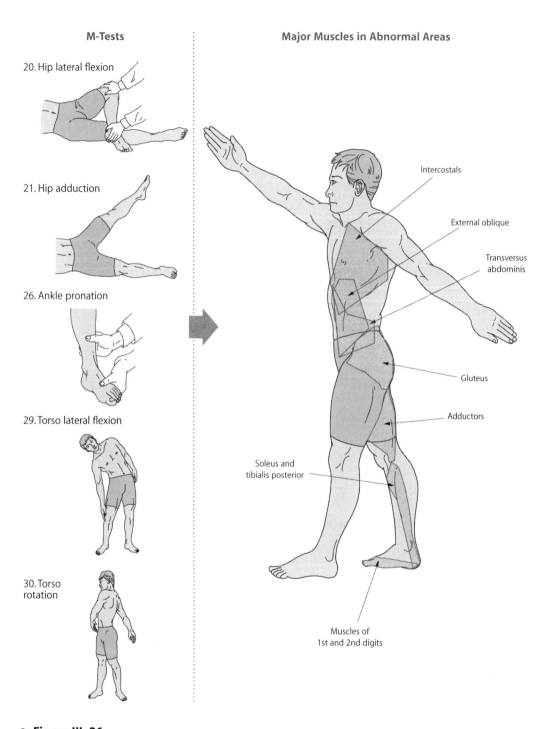

20. Hip lateral flexion

21. Hip adduction

26. Ankle pronation

29. Torso lateral flexion

30. Torso rotation

Intercostals

External oblique

Transversus abdominis

Gluteus

Adductors

Soleus and tibialis posterior

Muscles of 1st and 2nd digits

● **Figure III–26**

STEP **3** **Select the Acupuncture Points to Treat**   ANTERIOR UPPER BODY

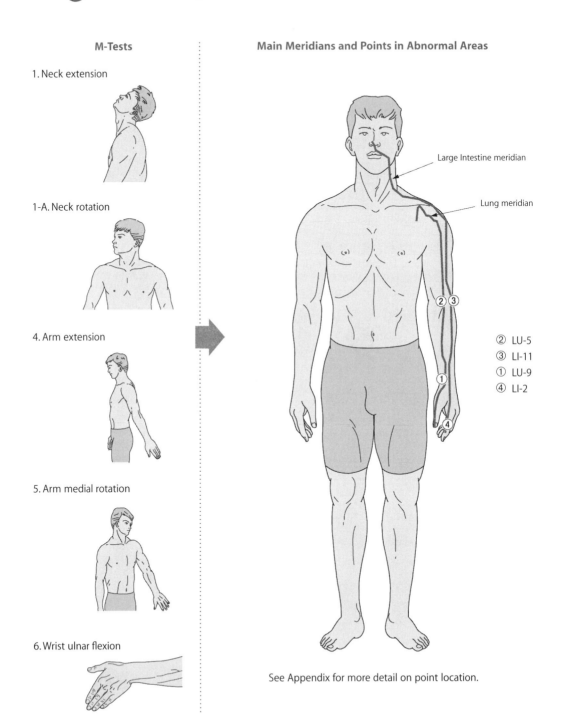

M-Tests

1. Neck extension

1-A. Neck rotation

4. Arm extension

5. Arm medial rotation

6. Wrist ulnar flexion

Main Meridians and Points in Abnormal Areas

Large Intestine meridian

Lung meridian

② ③

② LU-5
③ LI-11
① LU-9
④ LI-2

①

④

See Appendix for more detail on point location.

● **Figure III–27**

STEP **3**   **Select the Acupuncture Points to Treat**   POSTERIOR UPPER BODY |||

M-Tests	Main Meridians and Points in Abnormal Areas

2. Neck flexion

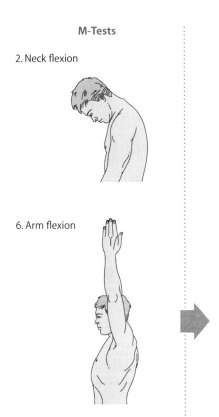

6. Arm flexion

7. Arm lateral rotation

13. Wrist radial flexion

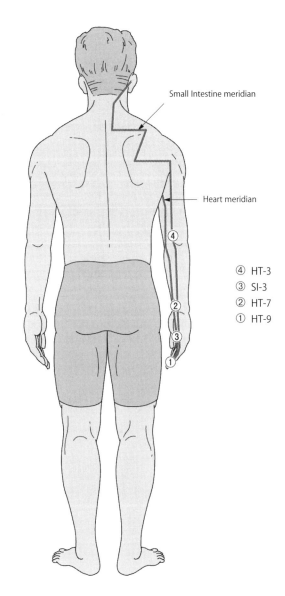

Small Intestine meridian

Heart meridian

④ HT-3
③ SI-3
② HT-7
① HT-9

See Appendix for more detail on point location.

● **Figure III–28**

STEP ❸ **Select the Acupuncture Points to Treat**   LATERAL UPPER BODY

M-Tests	Main Meridians and Points in Abnormal Areas

3. Neck lateral flexion

8. Arm horizontal flexion

9. Elbow flexion

14. Wrist flexion

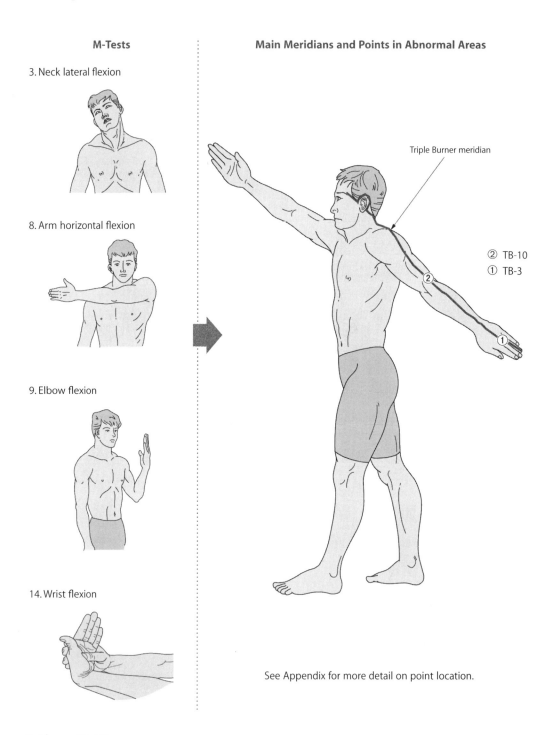

Triple Burner meridian

② TB-10
① TB-3

See Appendix for more detail on point location.

● **Figure III–29**

STEP **3** **Select the Acupuncture Points to Treat**   MEDIAL UPPER BODY   III

M-Tests	Main Meridians and Points in Abnormal Areas

3. Neck lateral flexion

10. Arm horizontal extension

11. Elbow extension

15. Wrist extension

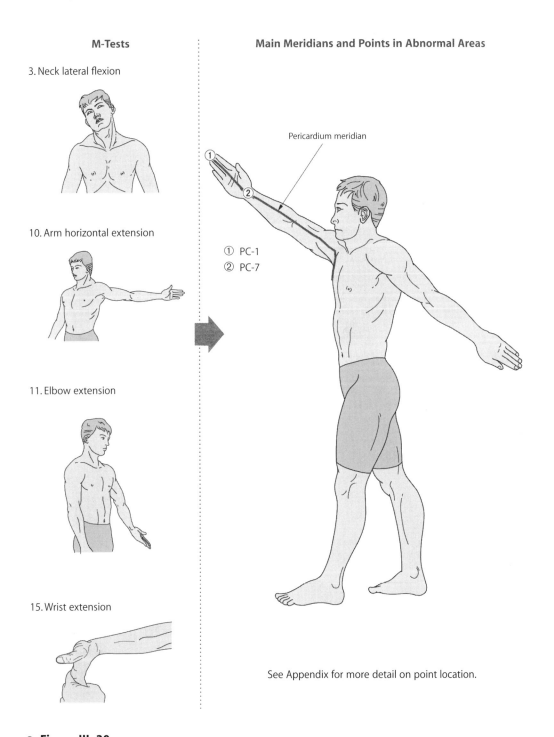

Pericardium meridian

① PC-1
② PC-7

See Appendix for more detail on point location.

● **Figure III–30**

STEP ③ **Select the Acupuncture Points to Treat**   ANTERIOR LOWER BODY

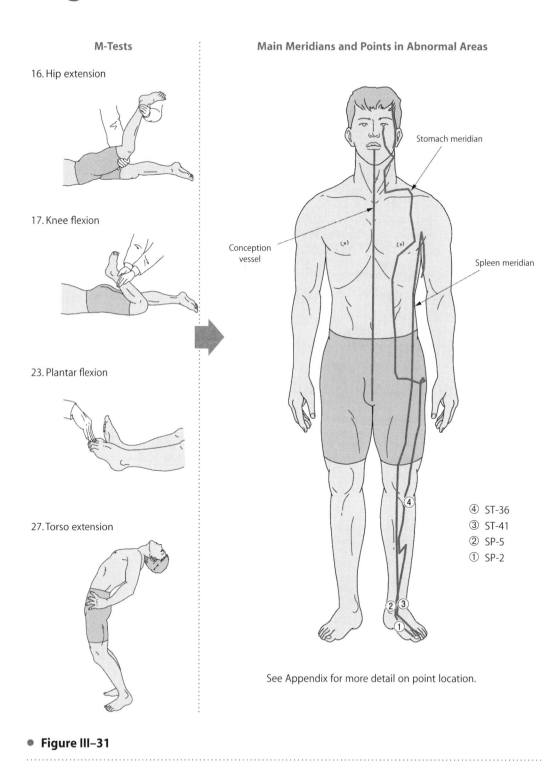

M-Tests

16. Hip extension

17. Knee flexion

23. Plantar flexion

27. Torso extension

Main Meridians and Points in Abnormal Areas

Stomach meridian

Conception vessel

Spleen meridian

④ ST-36
③ ST-41
② SP-5
① SP-2

See Appendix for more detail on point location.

● **Figure III–31**

STEP  **Select the Acupuncture Points to Treat**   POSTERIOR LOWER BODY |||

M-Tests	Main Meridians and Points in Abnormal Areas

M-Tests

18. Hip flexion

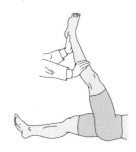

19. Knee and hip flexion

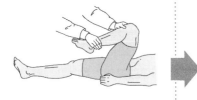

24. Dorsiflexion

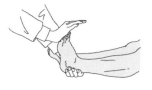

28. Torso flexion

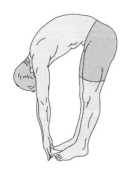

Main Meridians and Points in Abnormal Areas

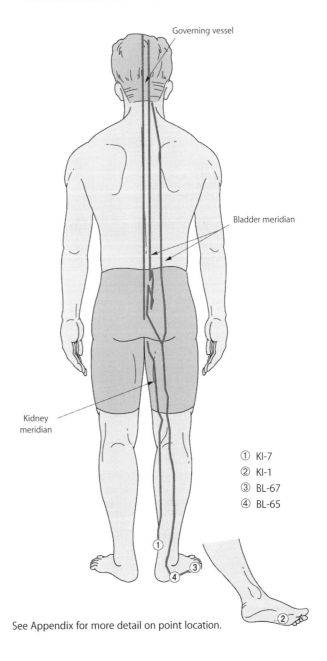

Governing vessel

Bladder meridian

Kidney meridian

① KI-7
② KI-1
③ BL-67
④ BL-65

See Appendix for more detail on point location.

● **Figure III–32**

STEP **3** **Select the Acupuncture Points to Treat**   LATERAL LOWER BODY

M-Tests

20. Hip external rotation

21. Hip adduction

25. Ankle supination

29. Torso lateral flexion

30. Torso rotation

Main Meridians and Points in Abnormal Areas

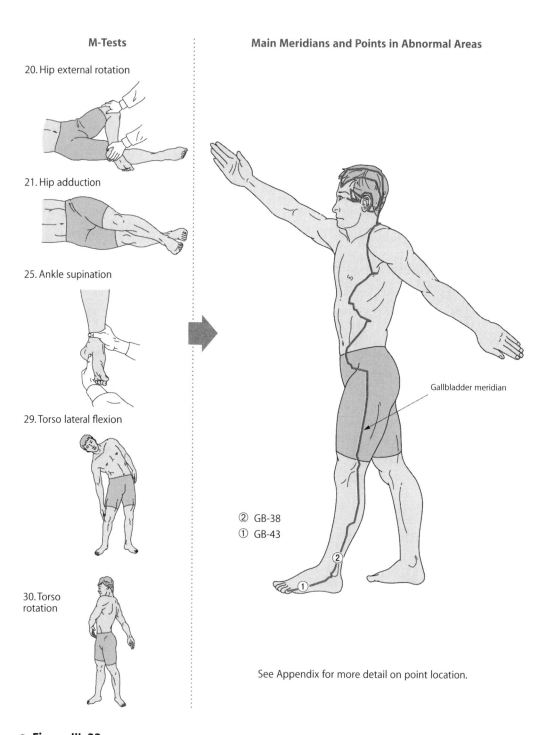

Gallbladder meridian

② GB-38
① GB-43

See Appendix for more detail on point location.

● **Figure III–33**

STEP ❸ **Select the Acupuncture Points to Treat**   LATERAL LOWER BODY |||

M-Tests

20. Hip external rotation

22. Hip abduction

26. Ankle pronation

29. Torso lateral flexion

30. Torso rotation

Main Meridians and Points in Abnormal Areas

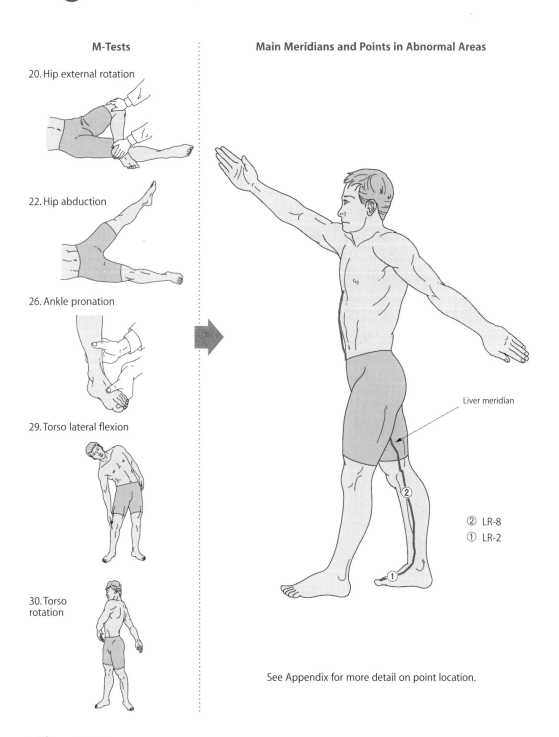

Liver meridian

② LR-8
① LR-2

See Appendix for more detail on point location.

● **Figure III–34**

STEP **4** **Confirm the effect of the points**

Apply finger pressure successively to the points selected in Step **3**, as the patient performs the problem movement, to determine whether there is an improvement in the movement or the symptom. If there is no change or improvement on pressing the first point, the other points and their related abnormal areas are pressed one point at a time to see if there is any improvement. If there is no change at all with finger pressure on any of the points, the patient should be referred for orthopedic examination. This procedure applies to all M-Tests.

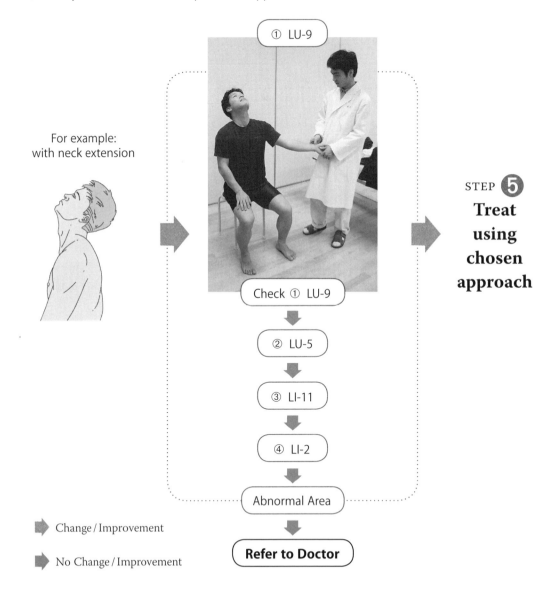

For example:
with neck extension

① LU-9

Check ① LU-9

② LU-5

③ LI-11

④ LI-2

Abnormal Area

Refer to Doctor

STEP **5**

Treat using chosen approach

Change / Improvement

No Change / Improvement

● **Figure III–35**

STEP **5** **Treat using chosen approach**   STRETCHING ANTERIOR ASPECT |||

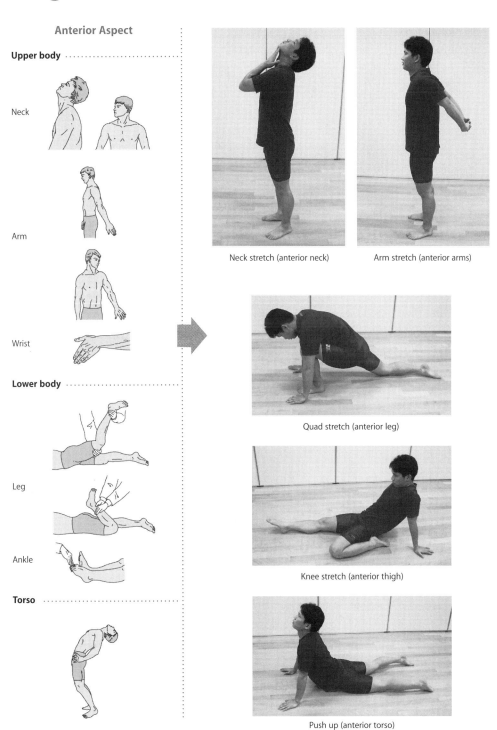

Anterior Aspect

Upper body

Neck

Arm

Wrist

Lower body

Leg

Ankle

Torso

Neck stretch (anterior neck)

Arm stretch (anterior arms)

Quad stretch (anterior leg)

Knee stretch (anterior thigh)

Push up (anterior torso)

● **Figure III–36**

STEP **5** **Treat using chosen approach**   STRETCHING POSTERIOR ASPECT

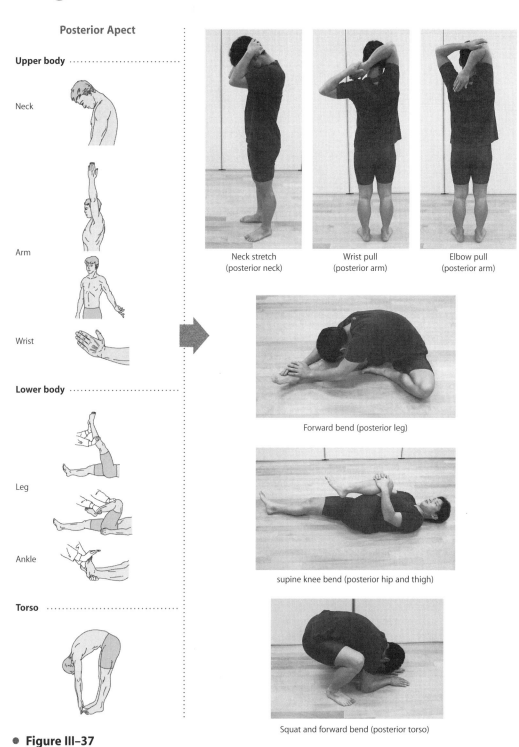

Posterior Apect

Upper body

Neck

Arm

Wrist

Lower body

Leg

Ankle

Torso

Neck stretch
(posterior neck)

Wrist pull
(posterior arm)

Elbow pull
(posterior arm)

Forward bend (posterior leg)

supine knee bend (posterior hip and thigh)

Squat and forward bend (posterior torso)

● **Figure III–37**

STEP **⑤** **Treat using chosen approach**   STRETCHING LATERAL ASPECT   III

Lateral Apect

Upper body

Neck

| LATERAL | MEDIAL |

Arm

Wrist

Lower body

Leg

Ankle

Torso

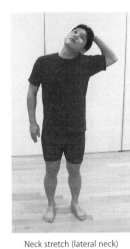

Neck stretch (lateral neck)

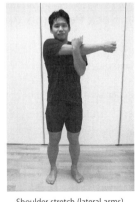

Shoulder stretch (lateral arms)

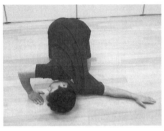

Arm stretch (medial arm)

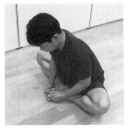

Knees to side (medial thigh)

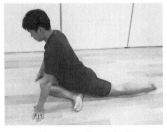

Pidgeon pose (lateral thigh)

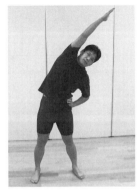

Side stretch (lateral torso)

● **Figure III–38**

☕ Coffee Break

Low Back Pain and the Big Toe

Mukaino Yoshito, M.D., Professor of the Faculty of Sports Science,
Fukuoka University

I was giving a lecture on sports medicine at a certain college, and, when I finished talking about acupuncture and moxibustion, a young judo wrestler came up to the podium asking me to examine his low back pain. Every time I teach there, several athletes come up to get my treatment and this had become something of a tradition.

I performed the M Tests on him, and, as shown in the figure below, adding stress with movement 16 on the right and movement 27 aggravated his low back pain. In other words, the low back pain seemed to be caused by restriction in extension of the anterior aspect. In addition, he had a mild pulling sensation when adding stress with movement 10 on the left. This finding indicated a restriction in extending the medial aspect of the left arm. I had him assume a prone position again and performed movement 16 on the right, as I successively pressed points along the Stomach and Spleen meridians on the anterior aspect. When I pressed SP-2 on the medial aspect of the big toe, the pain associated with the movement was relieved the most.

The abnormal sensation accompanying movement 10 with the left arm indicated a restriction in extending the Pericardium meridian (medial aspect of arm). I had the patient sit up and successively pressed points on the Pericardium meridian as he performed movement 10 with his left arm. He said the pulling sensation was the least when I pressed PC-7. So I had him stand up and repeat movement 27 as I pressed on his right SP-2 and left PC-7, and he no longer felt the low back pain. It seemed that these two points were the key to alleviating his low back pain.

| 16 right | 27 | 10 left | SP-2 | PC-7 |

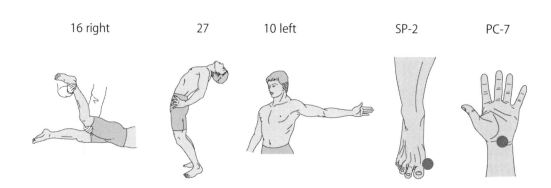

I asked him, "You have been putting some strain on your big toe, haven't you?" And he started to explain his judo form to me. He often supported his body with his left pivoting foot and stepped forward with his right to grapple with his opponent. This puts so much pressure onto his right foot that his big toe often digs into the mat. At the same time, he often used his left hand to powerfully pull his opponent toward him. Based on the effect that the above two points had, I realized that the excessive strain from this judo wrestler's moves was directly reflected in these points.

SP-2 and PC-7 are one of the five-phase point combinations I use from time to time. These point combinations often show me the effect of athletes' movements on their bodies.

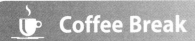

Coffee Break

The Effect of Strengthening Abdominal Muscles

Mukaino Yoshito, M.D., Professor of the Faculty of Sports Science, Fukuoka University

Once a female soccer player came to my clinic complaining that a muscle tear in her right calf was taking forever to heal. She said that her anterior thigh hurt when she sprinted, and she pleaded that I do something because an important match was coming up. So I performed the M-Test movements for the anterior, posterior, and lateral thigh, but none of the movements elicited any pain. Furthermore, there was not even tenderness when I pressed the place that she said had the pain. If the muscle tear had actually not healed, the M-Test movements would certainly have revealed an abnormality, and usually an injured area is quite tender. The fact that there was no abnormality at all indicated that the muscle tear had healed, or had never torn in the first place. So why then was there pain?

In situations like this there is always an underlying cause for the pain. So I asked her, "What do you do when the pain prevents you from running?" She replied that she had been doing exercises to strengthen her abdominal muscles everyday without fail since she had the muscle tear. Exercising the abdominal muscles places a strain on the anterior aspect of the body. I had a hunch that the pain in her anterior thigh was related to this. So I had her lie on her stomach and lift her head off the table a little, to add some stress to her abdominal area, and then performed movement 16 on the right (see figure below). This reproduced the pain that she had been feeling when she ran.

16 right

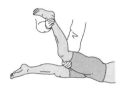

Thus it seemed that the key point for treatment lay in her abdominal muscles. So I had her lie on her back and pressed on her abdomen; she reported strong pain in the abdomen. I did some acupuncture on the most tender points in her abdomen and repeated the test with the above movement. She told me it did not cause pain this time. The next day she came to the clinic to give me a report: "I can run all out now, and I can give my best in the game," she said.

Placing excessive strain on other parts of the body before the injury to the right thigh had healed probably created another imbalance in movement. Even after the injury had healed, this imbalance had most likely continued to affect her performance. We can discover even the most unlikely causes of pain if we listen carefully to the athlete's story, and use a little imagination in how we apply these tests. ●

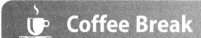

Coffee Break

Acupuncture Points for Pitching Curves

Miyazaki Shogo, Licensed Acupuncturist of the Faculty of Sports Science, Fukuoka University

One day I was at a ball field doing some research when I saw a pitcher practicing who repeatedly cocked his head with a quizzical expression. When I asked him what was going on, he told me that his curve ball, which was his forte, was not curving well. I asked him to show me how he threw it. He gripped the ball with his thumb and index finger (see figure below) and released the ball as he supinated his arm. I was convinced that he had a restriction in the anterior aspect of his arm. I therefore had the pitcher supinate his arm, and sure enough, he felt some tension with the movement. I just happened to have two intradermal needles (press tacks) with me, so I put them in LI-4 and LI-11, telling him that "these are points for throwing curves." (Of course, there are no such things.) I had him pitch curve balls again, and suddenly his touch had returned, and the pitches landed in the catcher's mitt where he intended. The pitcher exclaimed, "Wow, that's incredible!" and kept pitching as if to confirm this change.

A few days later another pitcher came up to me and asked, "Uhh, do you know if there are points for a fork ball?" ●

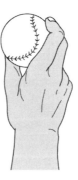

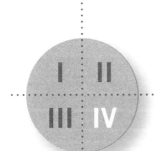

SECTION IV

Case Studies

CHAPTER 1

· ·

What Can be Achieved through the Meridian Test?

Mukaino Yoshito, M.D.

A. What is the Meridian Test?

MOVEMENTS OF THE BODY, from the simplest actions to sports activities, are comprised of multi-joint and multi-axial motions. In modern medicine the movement of individual joints and muscles are analyzed in detail, but the relationships of multi-joint and multi-axial motions have not been analyzed. Analysis of this type of movement is made possible, however, by applying the concept of meridians. A large number of acupuncture points are distributed over the body from the head down to the tip of the toes, on both arms and legs. The meridians are conceived as a system of pathways that connect the acupuncture points in a vertical axis. These meridians or pathways consist of the twelve regular meridians and another eight known as the Extraordinary vessels. The Meridian Test, or M-Test for short, is a physical assessment tool for quickly and accurately determining the reciprocal relationship of joints and muscles and possible dysfunctions with movements that stretch the meridians.

B. Features of the Meridian Test

1. The basic movements that stretch specific meridians are foundational movements for various complex movements.

2. One can determine which movements are strained or abnormal by compiling the results of the M-Test movements.

3. Strains or abnormalities that result from various sports can be analyzed simply.

139

4. Even for the same sport, the different locations of strain and abnormalities arising from each individual's form and unique misalignments can be identified.

5. The result of the assessment directly indicates the treatment required at that time.

6. The M-Test can be used to evaluate the results of treatment so that the treatment strategy can be easily reconsidered.

C. What Can be Achieved by Application of the Meridian Test

I. Conditioning

1. Abnormalities and fatigue in areas of which one is unaware can be quickly and accurately assessed.

2. When performed before or during competition, abnormalities of which one is unaware can be checked and corrected. In other words, stretching and massage can be done according to one's condition each day.

3. By making a habit of performing the M-Tests before each event, one can see the difference in abnormal areas when one has a good day and a bad day. Thus one can discover which areas need to be stretched or massaged to improve conditioning.

4. In situations where hard workouts are repeated, e.g., in training camp, one can discover the location of abnormalities of which one is unaware. Applying specific countermeasures to remedy these abnormalities can prevent injuries.

5. Since fatigue can be diminished, hard workouts can be performed more efficiently, which will increase the effect of the workout.

II. Performance

1. By using the M-Test, one can start to recognize the relationship between the characteristic form of each sport and the load placed on the meridians. Thus one can predict what kind of countermeasures will be necessary.

2. If acupuncture, stretching, and massage are performed in response to the M-Test results, the synergistic movement of the joints and muscles involved in the movement can be facilitated so that one can move the body just as one envisions.

3. Facilitating synergistic movement reduces fatigue in the mind and body and makes it possible to maintain one's abilities and perform optimally. For example:

a. The accuracy of the serve in tennis can be increased without a decrease in speed.

b. The speed of a pitch in baseball can be increased, and the fatigue with the same number of pitches decreased. The decrease in pitch speed can be prevented, and one's control improved.

c. New records can be achieved in sports like swimming and throwing events (e.g., discus).

d. The success rate of shots can be increased in sports like basketball.

Figure IV–1 shows the results of a study comparing pitching performance in baseball with and without acupuncture treatment, based on findings from the Meridian Test. In both instances, the pitcher was asked to throw sixty pitches as fast as he could. The difference in ball speed, and the integrated values of myograms in muscles around the shoulder, as well as the increase in the number of positive findings with the M-Test after pitching, were compared. The results show that, in the pitching that was done after treatment, the ball speed increased and the myogram values for the biceps brachii and triceps brachii decreased markedly. The ball speed increased as more pitches were

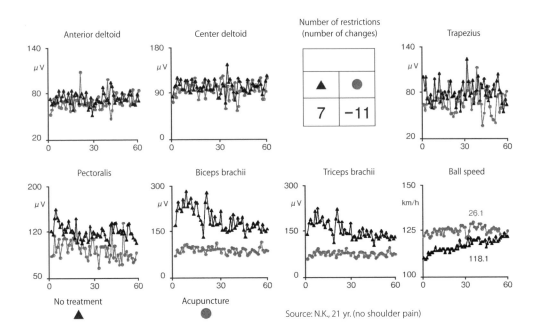

● **Figure IV–1**   The effect of M-Test on the integral values of myograms in muscles around the shoulder and ball speed

thrown in the pitching without treatment, and there was a concurrent decrease in the myogram values. In the pitching that was done after treatment, the ball speed remained constant from start to finish, but the speed remained faster than it was for those balls thrown without treatment. In the pitching without treatment, the number of positive findings in the M-Test increased after pitching. In the pitching that followed treatment, the number of positive findings decreased substantially, and there was less fatigue. This result suggests that the pitcher was able to move his body just as he intended.

III. Treatment

1. The selection of the meridians and points for treatment is quick because the positive findings reflect what needs to be treated.

2. Both the athlete and the practitioner can identify problematic movements (positive findings) so the athlete understands the aim of treatment.

3. Along with the abnormal sensations associated with problematic movement, the practitioner can note resistance to movement and right/left differences. In this way, the practitioner can accurately assess the results of treatment as well as any residual problems.

4. One can predict the relationship between the characteristic movements of a sport and the stress placed on the meridians. Even chronic problems can be resolved when this assessment is accurate.

5. The M-Test is a system for identifying imbalances or uneven strain patterns and correcting these imbalances. One sometimes finds that the cause of the pain lies in unexpected places. Also, the points to alleviate even chronic pain can be found by thorough examination. For example:

    a. Remarkable improvement in low back pain can be obtained by treating points on the arm.

    b. Stubborn knee pain in a long-distance runner can be alleviated by stimulating a combination of points on the posterior elbow and the anterior ankle.

    c. Pain in the abdomen during a 'smash' in a tennis game can be alleviated by stimulating points on the anterior leg.

6. Acupuncture points can be selected according to the principles of the five phases.

With the M-Test, the meridians and aspects of the body that need treatment are identified, and then the points that are effective in reducing the pain or restriction are located and treated. Even better results can be obtained by also treating meridians in what is called the 'generating cycle' of the five phases. I use five-phase point combinations in addition to the above-mentioned basic treatment strategy (treating the meridians indicated by positive findings). Treating five-phase points on the opposite side of meridians in a generating cycle serves to counterbalance the treatment on the affected areas and meridians. The five-phase points are all located on distal aspects of the arms and legs (on or below the elbow or knees) and serve to balance the whole body. There are only ten five-phase point combinations in my approach, so anyone can easily memorize them for this purpose. I have found this approach especially effective in treating athletes.

For example, if there is a restriction in the medial leg on the right, points on the Liver meridian (wood) on the right side are indicated for treatment. In the generating cycle of the five phases, the Heart and the Pericardium meridians (fire) follow the Liver meridian. The five-phase point combination for the wood and fire meridians is LR-2, HT-9, and PC-9. Thus, in addition to treating LR-2 on the right, HT-9 and PC-9 on the left wrist are treated to enhance the effect of treatment. There need not be any finding associated with the meridians that follow in the generating cycle. These meridians have a synergistic relationship that reinforce and consolidate one another.

Below is a table that shows my five-phase point combinations.

MERIDIANS	TREATMENT POINTS
Yin	
Wood (Liver) and fire (Heart, Pericardium)	LR-2, HT-9, PC-9
Fire (Heart, Pericardium) and earth (Spleen)	HT-7, PC-7, SP-2
Earth (Spleen) and metal (Lung)	SP-5, LU-9
Metal (Lung) and water (Kidney)	LU-5, KI-7
Water (Kidney) and wood (Liver)	KI-1, LR-8
Yang	
Wood (Gallbladder) and fire (Small Intestine, Triple Burner)	GB-38, SI-3, TB-3
Fire (Small Intestine, Triple Burner) and earth (Stomach)	SI-8, TB-10, ST-41
Earth (Stomach) and metal (Large Intestine)	ST-45, LI-11
Metal (Large Intestine) and water (Bladder)	LI-2, BL-67
Water (Bladder) and wood (Gallbladder)	BL-65, GB-43

● **Table IV–1** Five-phase point combinations

My colleagues and I have found these particular point combinations to be very effective. Nevertheless, five-phase points have been used since antiquity and many approaches have been utilized. Therefore, the use of five-phase points is by no means limited to those in this table.

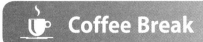

Acupuncture Points for Increasing the Batting Average

Miyazaki Shogo, Licensed Acupuncturist of the Faculty of Sports Science, Fukuoka University

The ball that baseball pitchers throw reaches the catcher's mitt in only 0.4 seconds if the speed of the pitch is 150 kilometers an hour (94 mph). In this very brief instant, the batter must determine the nature of the pitch and try to hit it. In this world of ball players where one must make instantaneous choices, there are many who receive treatment or 'training' for their eyes so that they can see the ball better.

Acupuncture can help ball players do this. Even if they experience no symptoms in their neck or shoulders, there are many ball players who have compromised movement in their neck and shoulders. When the neck doesn't turn well, not only is the ball harder to see, but also the batting form can start to deteriorate and the power in twisting the torso can be decreased. So we can test the neck movements of batters and help the head turn to the left if it's a right-handed hitter, and to the right if it's a left-handed hitter. This increases their field of vision and makes the ball easier to see. When I give ball players a treatment before a game, I always check their neck movements and treat them accordingly with the expectation that this will increase their batting averages. ●

. . . .

CHAPTER 2

Various Sports

A. Baseball

by Miyazaki Shogo

THE SPORT OF BASEBALL consists of throwing, catching, hitting, and running. Among these, throwing is especially important, and just one throw can make the difference between winning and losing. The whole body has to be used efficiently to add velocity to the ball and to throw a powerful fastball, or to accurately throw a curveball. Nevertheless, the fatigue that accumulates from daily practice and baseball games inhibits the smooth functioning of all the joints from the legs to the waist, shoulder, and arm. This can cause a decline in performance and lead to injuries. In this section, we will examine the cases of an overhand pitcher who has a right shoulder injury, a sidearm pitcher who has left hip pain, and another sidearm pitcher who has a problem with decreasing pitching speed. I will present case studies of these pitchers, each of whom showed improvement after acupuncture based on the movement analysis of the Meridian Test ('M-Test').

● CASE NO. 1: PITCHER WITH SHOULDER PAIN

22-year-old male pitcher (overhand)

CHIEF COMPLAINT: Pain in anterior right shoulder

HISTORY: He had been pitching over 200 pitches a day for many days, and the pain began just a few days before our appointment.

145

M-Test positive findings (see M-Test Chart, p. 204)

ANTERIOR: None

POSTERIOR: Right shoulder pain increased by lateral rotation with flexed elbow (Fig. IV–2). Some resistance felt with 6 (flexion of right shoulder) and 7 (supination of right arm).

LATERAL: Some resistance felt with 8 (horizontal extension of right shoulder) and 14 (flexion of right wrist).

Assessment & Treatment

Positive findings for movements in Figure IV–2, and 6 and 7 in M-Test Findings Chart: restriction in stretching posterior aspect of right arm (right Heart and Small Intestine meridians)

  POINTS: SI-4, SI-5, SI-8, SI-9, SI-11 on right side
  HT-1, HT-3 on right side

Positive findings for movements 8 and 14 in the M-Test Findings Chart: restriction in stretching lateral aspect of right arm (right Triple Burner meridian)

  POINTS: TB-4, TB-5, TB-10, TB-15 on right side

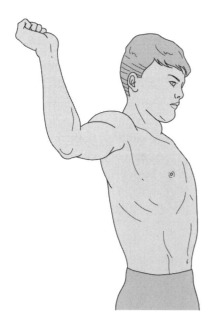

● **Figure IV–2**   External rotation of right shoulder (elbow flexed)

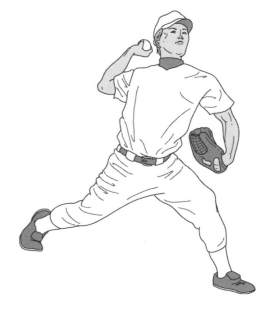

● **Figure IV–3**   Pitching form of right-handed pitcher (acceleration phase)

Progress

The same acupuncture treatment was performed twice and the pain almost disappeared.

Observations

It is instructive to consider the relationship between the meridians and the pitching form of a right-handed overhand pitcher. The sequence of the pitching movement begins with the wind-up, which puts the greatest stress on the pitching arm, and ends with the release of the ball. When we look at all aspects (meridians) of the arms and legs that are stretched by this motion, the right arm is like a bow and the posterior aspect (Heart and Small Intestine meridians) is stretched. Also, the anterior trunk is extended (Spleen and Stomach meridians) and the hips are simultaneously twisted such that the lateral aspect (Liver and Gallbladder meridians, and Girdle vessel) is stretched as well. Furthermore, the left arm, which acts like a rudder in transferring the power from the turned hips into the right arm, is stretched in the anterior aspect (Lung and Large Intestine meridians). The right leg that kicks the ground to move the body forward is stretched on the anterior aspect (Spleen and Stomach meridians), and the left leg that receives all the weight in the forward movement takes the load in the posterior aspect (Kidney and Bladder meridians).

In pitching, the characteristic movement of twisting and releasing the trunk delivers more power along with precise control. This is why it is important to check the pronation and supination of the arm (movements 5 and 7). For better discrimination, in some situations it is easier to check these movements with the elbow in 90 degree flexion. This is a case in which repeated pitching practice caused a restriction in extension of the right arm, which led to the symptom of right shoulder pain.

● CASE NO. 2: PITCHER WITH HIP PAIN

20-year-old male pitcher (sidearm)

CHIEF COMPLAINT: Pain in left hip

HISTORY: For the past three months, he had experienced hip pain when stepping forward to pitch.

M-Test positive findings (see M-Test Chart, p. 204)

ANTERIOR: 16 – resistance felt with extension of hip on right and left side

POSTERIOR: 18 – resistance felt with flexion of hip on right side

LATERAL: 20 – hip pain increased with external rotation of left hip

Assessment & Treatment

16: Restriction in stretching anterior aspects of both legs (right and left Spleen and Stomach meridians)

POINTS: ST-31, ST-32 bilateral
SP-9, SP-15 bilateral

18: Restriction in stretching posterior aspect of right leg (right Kidney and Bladder meridians)

POINTS: BL-36, BL-40, BL-57 on right side
KI-6, KI-10 on right side

20: Restriction in stretching lateral aspect of left leg (left Liver and Gallbladder meridians and the Girdle vessel)

POINTS: GB-25, GB-30, GB-31, GB-34 on left side
LR 8, LR-9, LR-13 on left side
GB-26 bilateral

Points on the Liver and Gallbladder meridians were selected by checking to see which ones were best at alleviating the symptom. In this way, the restriction that most aggravated the hip pain (the Patrick's test, or external rotation of left hip) was treated. This was followed by locating points on the Stomach and Spleen meridians to treat the restriction in the anterior aspect (16) of the left leg. Following treatment, the movement of stepping forward was checked for hip pain, and although it had improved, it had not completely disappeared. More points on the Stomach, Spleen, Bladder, and Kidney meridians were therefore added to treat the restriction in both the anterior and posterior aspects of the right leg (16 & 18). In addition, points affecting the central axis, the Girdle vessel points, and back *shu* points, were treated. This completely eliminated the hip pain when stepping forward.

Progress

In a game played one day after treatment, this player was able to pitch without being bothered by the hip pain, and in fact set a personal record for pitching speed.

Observations

Viewing the form of a sidearm pitcher (Fig. IV–4), the left leg that steps forward before the ball is released is flexed and stretched on the anterior aspect. The right pivoting leg is also stretched on the anterior aspect. In addition to this stretch on the anterior leg, the right ankle and toes are flexed forcefully, so there is a stretch in the posterior ankle as well. Also, since sidearm and underarm pitchers must twist their bodies more forcefully than overhand pitchers, there is a greater

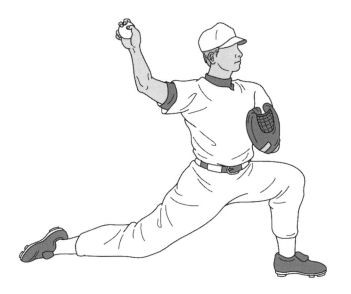

● **Figure IV–4** Pitching form of side-throwing pitcher

stress on the lateral aspects (Gallbladder and Liver meridians and the Girdle vessel). Furthermore, there is additional stress on the lateral and medial aspects of the forward leg in order to stabilize the knee and prevent it from moving outward with the twisting motion of the torso.

● CASE NO. 3: PITCHER WITH REDUCED PITCHING SPEED

19-year-old male pitcher (sidearm)

CHIEF COMPLAINT: Pitching speed decreases with repeated pitching

M-Test positive findings (see M-Test Chart, p. 204)

ANTERIOR: None

POSTERIOR: 18 – resistance felt with flexion of hip on right and left

LATERAL: 30 – resistance felt with rotation of torso to left

> Comparing the findings before and after pitching, resistance increased for 4 (extension of left shoulder) and 10 (horizontal flexion of left shoulder).

Assessment & Treatment

18: Restriction in stretching posterior aspects of both legs (right and left Kidney and Bladder meridians)

POINTS: BL-36, BL-40, BL-57 bilateral
KI-6, KI-10 bilateral

30: Restriction in stretching lateral aspect of right leg (right Gallbladder meridian and Girdle vessel)

POINTS: GB-25, GB-30, GB-31, GB-34 on right side
GB-26 bilateral

Intradermal needles (Seirin press tacks) were retained in the above points.

Progress

In this case, I had the pitcher throw 100 pitches in a row as fast as he could and recorded the speed of each pitch; this was repeated on another day with intradermal needles taped in place over the above points. Also, I performed the M-Test before and after each trial to compare the results.

In the trial without needles (Fig. IV–5a) the speed of the ball began to decrease gradually after about 50 throws. In the M-Test preceding the trial, resistance was felt subjectively on the posterior legs (Bladder and Kidney meridians) and lateral trunk (Liver and Gallbladder meridians and Girdle vessel). In the M-Test conducted after the trial, there was an increase in resistance felt on the medial (Pericardium meridian) and anterior aspect (Lung and Large Intestine meridians) of the pitching arm.

In the trial with needles in place (Fig. IV–5b) the speed of the ball remained stable and decreased very little. Also, the resistance in the pitching arm noted before starting showed almost no increase after 100 pitches.

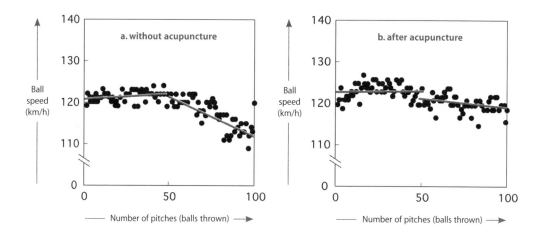

● **Figure IV–5**   Changes in pitching speed after acupuncture

IV

Observations

In this case, the fatigue that accumulated in the lower half of the body as the number of pitches increased is thought to have added to the strain on the pitching arm. This is most likely what led to the decline in pitching performance. It seems probable that the acupuncture treatment targeting the compromised movements identified by the M-Test reduced the accumulation of fatigue and prevented the decline in pitching speed. Balanced movement in the entire body can be achieved when the movements of individual joints are facilitated by this method. This obviously leads to better performance.

B. Track

1) Long-Distance Running

by Noguchi Hiroko

Long-distance running is a simple sport which does not require any equipment or much technique, but neither is it just a back and forth movement of the arms and legs. It requires twisting of the torso and stability. It is a whole-body sport involving a chain of movement, from the arm and torso down to the legs, which is repeated for a long time. Thus it is important that each part of the body moves smoothly, especially to run the last half of the race with an efficient form and minimum fatigue. In the case discussed below, a long-distance runner with knee pain was assessed and treated based on the M-Test to improve performance.

● CASE NO. 1: LONG-DISTANCE RUNNER WITH KNEE PAIN

21-year-old female runner (running career: 6 years)

CHIEF COMPLAINT: Pain in right knee

HISTORY: She ran a hilly course several days in a row at a training camp; the amount of practice was also more than usual, and she started to experience knee pain.

M-Test positive findings (see M-Test Chart, p. 204)

ANTERIOR: 1 right and left, 4 right and left, 16 right and left, 23 right, 27 right and left

POSTERIOR: None

LATERAL: 3 right, 20 right and left, 26 right, 29 right

(The pain was especially pronounced with movements 23 and 26.)

Assessment & Treatment

1 & 4: Lung meridian (LU-1, LU-5)

3: Triple Burner meridian (TB-10)

16 & 23: right Stomach meridian (ST-36, ST-41)

20 & 26: right Gallbladder meridian (GB-38, GB-41)

27: Conception vessel (CV-12)

29: Girdle vessel (GB-26)

Progress

The knee pain improved after the first treatment. It completely disappeared after one month of treatment, given twice a week.

Observations

The running action of the legs can be roughly divided into two phases: One is the stepping phase, between the time the foot lands and kicks off, and the other is the swinging phase, when it comes forward. In the stepping phase, the hip joint transitions from flexion and external rotation (Kidney, Bladder, and Liver meridians) to extension and medial rotation (Spleen, Stomach, and Gallbladder meridians). Also, the ankle joint transitions from slight dorsiflexion and eversion (Kidney, Bladder, and Liver meridians) to plantar flexion and inversion (Spleen, Stomach, and Gallbladder meridians). The aspects of the body that are stretched during the swinging phase are the opposite of the stepping phase (Fig. IV–6). As for movement of the arms, they transition from shoulder flexion (Heart and Small Intestine merid-

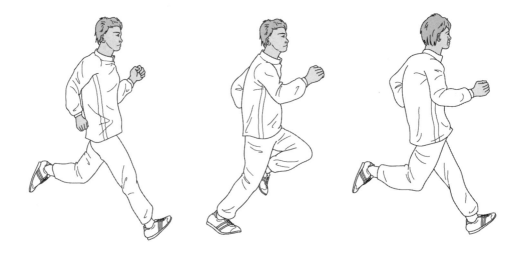

● **Figure IV–6**   Extension phase and flexion phase (right leg)

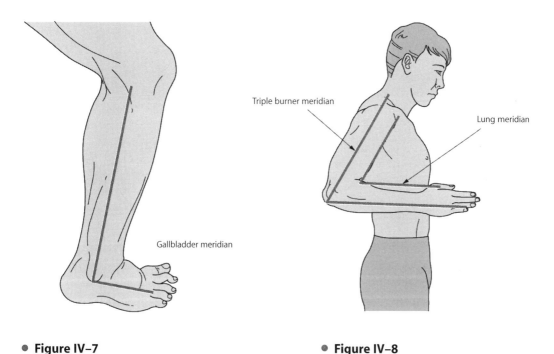

Triple burner meridian

Lung meridian

Gallbladder meridian

● **Figure IV–7**

● **Figure IV–8**

ians) and shoulder extension (Lung and Large Intestine meridians) with the elbows flexed. In order for the arm-swinging motion to go smoothly, however, there must also be flexibility in the scapular area (Small Intestine meridian) and interscapular area (Bladder meridian). In the case of long-distance running, the stress on parts of the body repeatedly alternates, so performance depends on how relaxed a runner can remain from start to finish. In the above case, there was strong eversion in the ankle when the feet landed, and it seems that the stress on the anterior (Stomach meridian) and lateral (Gallbladder meridian) aspects led to the knee pain. In the upper body, the right arm swung further away from the side and pulled back further in the latter half of the race, which stressed the lateral (Triple Burner meridian) and anterior (Lung meridian) aspects. Thus it was seen how one imbalance led to other imbalances through the rest of the body.

A significant relief in pain was achieved by treating the five-phase combination of ST-41 and TB-10. (The Stomach meridian, associated with the symptom of knee pain, is earth, and the Triple Burner meridian is fire. Fire and earth are in a generating relationship.) I continued to perform M-Test assessments on this runner periodically. The loss of speed in the latter half of the race decreased and she started to improve her time. Both for improving performance and preventing injury, it is important to balance the whole body on a daily basis in terms of muscle fatigue, muscle strength, and flexibility.

2) Sprinting

by Fukazawa Hiroki

In track events, many of which are entirely about how fast one runs a given distance, the outcome depends on how efficiently and quickly one is able to perform the movements of running. To run, one must swing the arms, twist the torso, and kick the ground to bring the leg forward (Fig. IV–9). This movement is simply repeated back and forth on each side, but even this simple movement demands coordination of the whole body. In other words, the arms, legs, and torso must be positioned in a balanced way within this sequence of movements. In the case below, leg pain from running was assessed and treated based on the M-Test.

● CASE NO. 2: SPRINTER WITH LEG PAIN

18-year-old female runner (student)

CHIEF COMPLAINT: Pain in posterior right leg

HISTORY: The pain started about two months ago while running. She felt the pain especially in the posterior leg when stretching. Also, her calf muscle felt tense and heavy when she started to run, and was slightly swollen. She had been participating in college track team practice after just recently graduating high school.

M-Test positive findings (see M-Test Chart, p. 204)

ANTERIOR: 1-A left, 16 right, 27 right and left

POSTERIOR: 2 right and left, 18 right and left

LATERAL: 3 right and left, 20 right

Assessment & Treatment

1-A: left Large Intestine meridian (LI-4)

27: right and left Stomach meridian (ST-36)

2: left Small Intestine meridian (SI-8)

16: right Stomach meridian (ST-41, earth) with five-phase combination (TB-10, fire)

18: right and left Kidney meridian (KI-1, water) with five-phase combination (LR-8, wood)

3: right and left Gallbladder meridian (GB-21)

20: right Liver meridian (LR-2)

Seirin red (0.16mm) 30mm needles were inserted just a few millimeters in each of the above points and the needles were not retained.

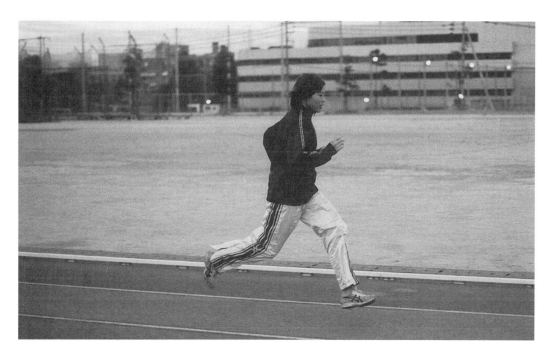

● **Figure IV–9**

Progress

The pain in the right posterior leg decreased after the treatment, and it was at a level that did not bother her while running. After four more treatments in six days, the pain disappeared. Also, there was no more tension in the calf muscle or pain with stretching.

Observations

This student was at a high level of competition, being a frequent competitor in high school track meets, but her training environment underwent a big change from high school to college. The track at her high school was dirt, but the track at her college consisted of an all-weather material called Tartan. She said that it felt harder than any track she had experienced in high school. When the landing surface is hard, the impact on the feet and legs as a whole is correspondingly greater. This could add an extra stress on a body that is accustomed to running on dirt, and therefore pose a problem. It could also be a factor that she ran repeatedly on the Tartan college track right after the off-season when she was not yet in good shape.

Running places stress on the meridians on the anterior and posterior aspects of the body (Fig. IV–9). In terms of the legs, the anterior meridians are the Spleen and Stomach, and the posterior meridians are the Kidney and Bladder. Considering the acupuncture points that were most effective for this case, it seemed that the Stomach and Kidney meridians especially were under excessive stress. The reason LR-2 worked well to alleviate the restriction in movement 20 is probably because the impact on the foot had caused a problem around the right big toe, and this influenced the stretching movements of the medial aspect, which is governed by the Liver meridian.

Balance, and problems with the body during running, can be assessed and corrected by giving acupuncture based on the positive M-Test findings. This is a powerful tool for conditioning, and can help an athlete reach a higher level of performance.

3) Javelin Throw

by Miyazaki Shogo

The javelin throw involves a sequence of movements starting with the run-up, stepping, stopping, releasing, and follow-through. The javelin can be thrown the greatest distance by performing this sequence of movements precisely according to one's mental picture. For this to occur, all the joints from the foot, pelvis, shoulder, to the arm must move in a coordinated and efficient manner to transfer the force into the javelin. Smooth and coordinated movement is not possible, however, if there is fatigue or injury in any part of this chain. Below is a case of a javelin thrower with pain in the right shoulder and knee who won a place in an important competition because of assessment and treatment based on the M-Test.

● CASE NO. 3: JAVELIN THROWER WITH SHOULDER AND KNEE PAIN

22-year-old male

CHIEF COMPLAINT: Pain in the right shoulder and knee

M-Test positive findings (see M-Test Chart, p. 204)

ANTERIOR: None

POSTERIOR: 6 right (shoulder flexion); pain is aggravated
    7 right (arm supination); tension is felt

Assessment & Treatment

Findings 6 and 7 both indicate restrictions in stretching the right
    arm.
    POINTS: Right Small Intestine meridian (SI-3, SI-4, SI-8, SI-9 &
    SI-11)

Right Heart meridian (HT-1, HT-3)

Back *shu* points (BL-15, BL-27)

Front *mu* points (CV-14, CV-4)

Result

The pain diminished with one treatment and he was able to place in an important competition.

Observations

The relationship between the javelin thrower's form and the meridians can be understood by studying the figure of the throwing form at the release phase, the most significant stage for throwing the greatest distance (Fig. IV–10). The aspects (meridians) of the arms and legs that are stretched include the posterior aspect of the throwing arm (Heart and Small Intestine meridians), which is arched back. Also the torso, which is arched forward, is stretched in the anterior aspect (Spleen and Stomach meridians), as well as in the lateral aspect (Liver and Gallbladder meridians, and Girdle vessel) that is twisted strongly at the pelvis. The right leg that kicks the ground to propel the body forward is stretched on the anterior aspect (Spleen and Stomach meridians), while the left leg that comes to the front to catch the full weight of the body is stressed on the posterior aspect (Kidney and Bladder meridians).

The difference between this form and the throwing form of a pitcher (Table IV–2) involves three main components: the grip, the torso movement, and the step angle of the knee on the front leg. As for the grip, in baseball the first, second, and third fingers are used the most; in javelin throwing, the fourth and fifth fingers are used the most. Therefore in pitching, the stress goes to the anterior (Lung and Large Intestine) and medial (Pericardium) aspects, while in javelin throwing, the stress goes on the posterior (Heart and Small Intestine)

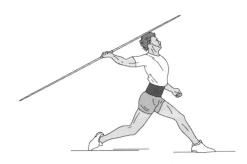

	Baseball	Javelin throwing
① Grip	1st, 2nd & 3rd fingers	4th & 5th fingers
② Torso movement	Twisting is essential	Arching is essential
③ Step angle of knee of front leg	Small	Large

● **Figure IV–10** Javelin throwing form (release phase)

● **Table IV–2** Difference between baseball and javelin throwing

and lateral (Triple Burner) aspects. As for the movement of the torso, arching is essential in pitching as well as in javelin throwing, but twisting of the torso is more important for generating power in the throw in pitching. Because of the differences in the run-up, the object thrown, and the aim in javelin throwing, the arching of the torso is more important for generating power in the throw. As for the angle of knee on the front leg, because the center of gravity must be kept low in pitching, the front knee is flexed quite a bit. In javelin throwing, the front leg must be kept stiff (knee extended) to stop the forward movement of the body.

If there is a restriction in any part of the body involved in the sequence of movements for javelin throwing, the coordination of the entire sequence is compromised. This can lead to a decline in performance as well as injury. The places where restrictions occur vary based on the individual's form or the way one practices, so it is recommended that treatment be given according to the M-Test findings. In the case above, the athlete practiced more intensively in preparation for competition, and this caused a restriction in stretching of the posterior aspect of the arm. This restriction, no doubt, was what caused the pain.

4) Long Jump

by Fukazawa Hiroki

In the long jump, athletes compete to see how far they can jump from the takeoff board after running as fast as they can down the approach runway. Gaining the greatest jump distance requires top speed and jumping power. Coordination of the whole body is crucial, even in the one motion of the takeoff jump, and the execution of this movement can make a big difference in the distance. Therefore, it is important to sprint down the approach runway and transfer this momentum smoothly into the takeoff in a balanced way with the movements of the arms, legs, and torso. Below is a case of a long jumper with pain in his leg from repeatedly practicing his takeoff. He was assessed and treated successfully using the M-Test.

● CASE NO. 4: LONG JUMP ATHLETE WITH KNEE PAIN

18-year-old male (student on the track team)

CHIEF COMPLAINT: Pain in the left knee

HISTORY: He noticed discomfort during running for two months, and then developed pain and discomfort, especially during the takeoff. Twice while riding a bicycle he experienced such discomfort in his knee that he had to stop pedaling.

M-Test positive findings (see M-Test Chart, p. 204)

ANTERIOR: 16 left, 17 left, 23 left, 27 left

POSTERIOR: 18 left

LATERAL: 20 left

Assessment & Treatment

ANTERIOR: 16 left (left Stomach meridian), left ST-41. Five-phase combination of earth and fire (Triple Burner and Small Intestine meridians): right TB-10 and right SI-8

ANTERIOR: 17 left (Stomach meridian on both sides), ST-36
    23 left (left Stomach meridian), ST-45
    27 left (Stomach front *mu* point), CV-12

POSTERIOR: 18 left (left Kidney meridian), left KI-1. Five-phase combination of water and wood (Liver meridian), left LR-8

LATERAL: 20 left (left Liver meridian), LR-2

    Seirin red (0.16mm) 30mm needles were inserted in each of the above points; the needles were not retained. Intradermal needles (Seirin press tacks) were retained in tender points over the sacroiliac joint.

Result

The discomfort and pain in the knee diminished immediately after the first treatment. Eight similar treatments were given over the subsequent month, and his complaint resolved completely. Also, retaining

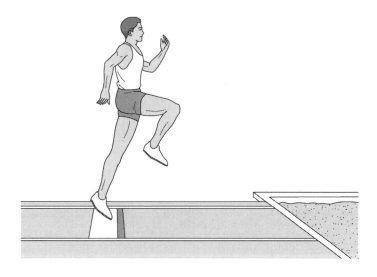

● **Figure IV–11**

intradermal needles in tender points over the sacroiliac joint was very effective in alleviating the pain when it was at its worst.

Observations

This is another case that is most likely related to a change in the training environment. The athlete's practice field in high school was dirt, but in college the grounds were an all-weather material called Tartan. Repeated practice of sprinting over the hard Tartan track in spiked shoes without shock absorbing soles caused his knee to take a greater impact than ever before. This also increased the strain on his legs as a whole, and probably this excessive strain led to an injury since he was accustomed to running on a softer surface. Another contributing factor could be that he used to run downhill about 10 kilometers once a week for practice while he was still in high school.

The anterior and posterior meridians are stretched in running. In the legs, the anterior meridians are the Spleen and Stomach and the posterior meridians are the Kidney and Bladder. Considering the points that were especially effective in the above case, it is obvious that excessive strain was placed on the Stomach and Kidney meridians. Also, the reason LR-2 was effective in treating finding 20 is probably because the impact of landing had caused a problem in the area of the right big toe and this affected the movement on the lateral aspect, which is governed by the Liver meridian.

Physical imbalances and problems during running can be assessed and corrected by giving acupuncture based on the positive M-Test findings. This is a useful tool for conditioning, and aids the athlete in attaining a higher level of performance.

C. Archery (Kyu-do)

by Miyazaki Shogo

In Kyu-do, the traditional art of archery in Japan, the act of shooting an arrow is divided into eight stages, called the 'eight stages of shooting' (*shaho hassetsu*). Although each stage may appear simple, all the muscles of the body must be used to maintain the correct posture, and it requires subtle adjustments. Performing this sequence of movements in a relaxed and efficient manner while maintaining a stable and correct posture contributes to hitting the target. Restrictions in various parts of the body that affect the movements of archery, however, can prevent one from executing the movements correctly as visualized. Over time, these restrictions can cause a decline in performance and even injury. Below is a case of pain in the left shoulder, low back, and left knee that was probably caused by the strain placed on the arms and legs by repeatedly practicing the movements of archery.

● CASE STUDY: ARCHER WITH SHOULDER, BACK, AND KNEE PAIN

Female archer in her fifties

CHIEF COMPLAINT: pain in the left shoulder, low back, and left knee

HISTORY: The pain appears after archery practice and competition

M-Test positive findings (see M-Test Chart, p. 204)

ANTERIOR: None

POSTERIOR: 6 left (shoulder flexion) aggravates the shoulder pain

LATERAL: 20 both sides (external rotation of hips) resistance is felt

Assessment & Treatment

6: Restriction in extension of posterior aspect of left arm (Small Intestine and Heart meridians)

POINTS: Heart meridian (left HT-1, HT-3, HT-7)
Small Intestine meridian (left SI-4, SI-5, SI-8, SI-9, SI-11)

20: Restriction in extension of medial aspect of both legs (Gallbladder and Liver meridians)

POINTS: Gallbladder meridian (bilateral GB-40, GB-39, GB-34, GB-31, GB-30, GB-25)

Liver meridian (bilateral LR-4, LR-8, LR-9, LR-13)

Gallbladder and Liver back *shu* points (bilateral BL-19, BL-18)

Gallbladder and Liver front *mu* points (bilateral GB-24, LR-14)

Girdle vessel (bilateral GB-26)

Result

Selecting effective points by confirming that they improved the above positive findings relieved the symptoms. But the symptoms reappeared whenever the amount of practice was increased or when she took part in many competitions. This aggravation is expected to continue, so treatments must be given repeatedly.

Observations

Among the sequence of movements in archery, I focused on the *kai* or 'drawing' stage because it is the most influential in hitting the target. Let us consider the relationship between the meridians and the posture in this stage of the Japanese archery form (Fig. IV–12).

The 'drawing' stage is one in which the bow is drawn fully like a full moon, so that it cannot be pulled or pushed any more. In this posture, it is necessary to use even force to push the bow with the left

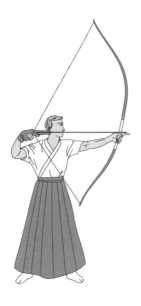

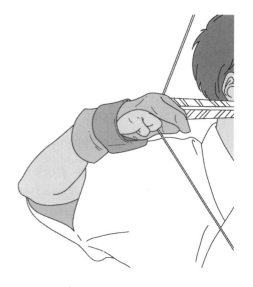

● **Figure IV–12** 'Drawing' form

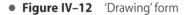

● **Figure IV–13** Grip of right hand

hand and draw the string with the right. Also, it is considered good form when the line connecting the two hands is perpendicular to the vertical line through the center of the torso. Considering the aspects (meridians) of the arms and legs that are extended in this posture, the right arm draws the bow while holding the arrow and the string with the thumb and middle finger (Fig. IV–13). This places a strong extension load on the medial (Pericardium) aspect of the right arm. The left arm grasps the bow firmly with the fourth and fifth fingers while pushing it forward, so the posterior aspect (Heart and Small Intestine) of the arm is extended. It is not easy to see, but the torso and legs bear various loads to maintain a stable and correct posture. In order to stabilize the legs and maintain the correct posture, one must draw the knees together and bring one's weight over the big toes. For this reason, the legs bear a load in the medial and lateral aspects.

When there is residual fatigue, or a buildup of fatigue during practice, these movements can be slightly off; the smooth coordination of the sequence of movements is thereby disturbed, which can influence the accuracy of the shots. Also, the loss of smooth coordination can itself become the cause of physical problems. In the above case, the strain of repeatedly practicing this sequence of archery movements caused a restriction in the posterior aspect of the arm and the lateral aspect of the leg, and this most likely caused pain in the left shoulder, low back, and left knee.

D. Judo (Wrestling)

by Ishizue Shinichi

There are certain throwing techniques in judo in which the opponent is pulled off balance and thrown forward or backward. Among the forward-throwing techniques are the shoulder throw, the sweeping hip throw, the inner thigh throw, and the body drop. In these techniques, the wrestler must pull the opponent forward and throw him by twisting his own body and pulling the hand grasping the opponent's sleeve in front and tripping him over his bent knee.

The throwing techniques of judo require good timing in pulling an opponent off balance and speed in executing the throw. The judo technique is effective when the sequence of movements involving the arms and legs and torso comes together smoothly.

Below is a case of low back pain that began after doing judo throws that was evaluated and treated based on the M-Test.

● CASE STUDY: JUDO WRESTLER WITH LOW BACK PAIN

48-year-old male (civil servant and judo instructor)

CHIEF COMPLAINT: low back pain on left side

HISTORY: This man began to experience low back pain on the left side two days earlier, after practicing with a student. The student was especially large, and the patient used the throwing technique of body drop, repeatedly throwing the student over his left side because he was left-handed. He thought that the back pain would resolve by itself, but it did not. Bending forward and sideways aggravated the pain.

M-Test positive findings (see M-Test Chart, p. 204)

ANTERIOR: 4 right (shoulder extension)

POSTERIOR: 18 left (hip flexion)
  28 (torso flexion)

LATERAL: 3 left (neck lateral flexion)
  29 left (torso lateral flexion)
  30 left (torso rotation)

Assessment & Treatment

3: left Triple Burner meridian (TB-10)
4: right Large Intestine meridian (LI-11)
18: left Kidney meridian (KI-7)
28: left Kidney meridian (KI-7)

29: left Gallbladder meridian (GB-38, GB-31)

30: left Gallbladder meridian (GB-26)

Intradermal needles (Seirin press tacks) were retained in the above points.

Result

The positive findings of the M-Test disappeared right after the treatment, and bending forward and sideways caused only slight back pain. The pain resolved completely the next day.

Observations

In the body drop of judo, one hand grasps the opponent's sleeve and pulls him forward. In so doing, the torso must be twisted quickly to effect the throw. The timing and speed of this twist determines the effectiveness of this technique (Fig IV–14). In this sequence of movements, the lateral aspect of the body (Gallbladder meridian) is strained (Fig IV–15) along with the anterior aspect of the arm (Lung and Large Intestine meridians), which must be extended while turning the wrist (Fig. IV–16).

Furthermore, once the weight of the opponent who has lost his balance comes over the left leg, which is bent, the left knee must be quickly extended to lift the opponent forward and upward to complete the throw. This puts stress on the medial posterior aspect (Kidney meridian) of the left leg (Fig. IV–17).

The most effective acupuncture points in this treatment were LI-11, for the restriction in stretching the anterior right leg, and KI-7, for the restriction in stretching the posterior left leg. Also, in judo throws, one must use the opponent's strength against him, get him off balance, and then execute the technique lightning fast. The speed of twisting one's body, especially, is crucial for the success of this technique. This makes it important to treat restrictions in the meridians on the side of the body, and to this end, GV-26 was very useful.

In this case, the patient repeatedly used the body drop throwing technique on a large opponent, grasping and throwing with his left hand, and this stressed certain aspects (meridians) to cause the low back pain. By performing acupuncture based on the findings of the M-Test, the strains involved in this throwing technique of judo were analyzed and successfully treated.

In recent years, judo has become an international sport and it is rare for a match to be decided by just one move. Nevertheless, the original appeal of judo lay in using a person's strength against him, making a quick move, and decisively winning by executing one good throw. Even if there are no symptoms, I believe it is important to adjust a wrestler's physical balance using the M-Test so that he can execute a technique decisively, and also avoid injury.

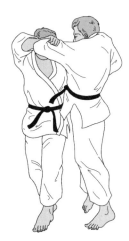

● **Figure IV–14**

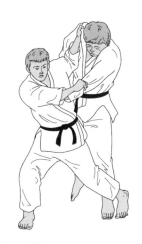

● **Figure IV–15**

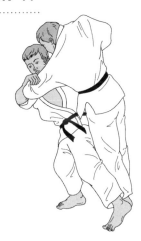

● **Figure IV–16**

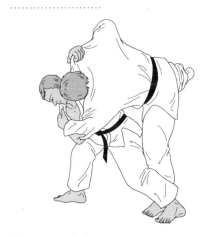

● **Figure IV–17**

E. Rugby

by Honda Tatsuro

In describing the sport of rugby one might say, "It's a rough contact sport over an oval-shaped ball that's hard to predict where it will roll." Players in rugby are divided into two contrasting positions: forwards and backs. Injuries are common since body contact with opponents is unavoidable during a game.

On the other hand, injuries due to overuse also occur quite often during practice. The cause of this type of injury is harder to pinpoint. Also, it is not uncommon to drop out of the team and cease practicing for a period due to injuries. Here I would like to present a case with symptoms that originated from the unique movements of rugby, and use the positive findings of the M-Test to analyze the condition.

● CASE STUDY: RUGBY PLAYER WITH LOW BACK PAIN

23-year-old male (position: back)

CHIEF COMPLAINT: low back pain

HISTORY: The day before I saw him, this player's low back suddenly began to hurt when he was practicing for a match, and he was no longer able to walk as usual. He said he felt nothing unusual when he began practice. During practice he practiced hits (running into the defenders while in possession of the ball), but he didn't suffer any strong direct impacts on his back.

M-Test positive findings (see M-Test Chart, p. 204)

ANTERIOR: ① 27 (extension of torso)

POSTERIOR: None

LATERAL: ② 29 left (torso lateral flexion)
   ③ 30 left (torso rotation)
   ④ 21 left and right (hip adduction)
   ⑤ 20 left (hip external rotation)

Assessment & Treatment

Since the majority of findings were on the lateral aspect, the treatment was done in the following order: lateral aspect ②, ③, ④, medial aspect ⑤, anterior aspect ①.

Since the findings ②, ③, and ④ were restrictions in the Gallbladder meridian, the following points were used: bilateral GB-38 (Fig. IV–18-5), bilateral GB-31 (Fig. IV–18-6) right, GB-30 (Fig. IV–18-7) right, GB-26 (Fig. IV–18-8).

Since the finding ⑤ was a restriction in the Liver meridian, the following point was used: left LR-9 (Fig. IV–18-9).

Since the finding ① was a restriction in the Stomach meridian, the following points were used: bilateral ST-41 (Fig. IV–18-1), bilateral ST-36 (Fig. IV–18-2), bilateral ST-32 (Fig. IV–18-3), bilateral ST-31 (Fig. IV–18-4).

Intradermal needles (Seirin press tacks) were retained in the above points. Also, the tight points on the lateral legs, hip, and lumbar area were massaged. After this, the M-Test was performed again to confirm the change in the above-listed movements.

Results

Following treatment, there was no more pain with the M-Test movements at issue. Furthermore, the player was able to play as usual in the game the following day.

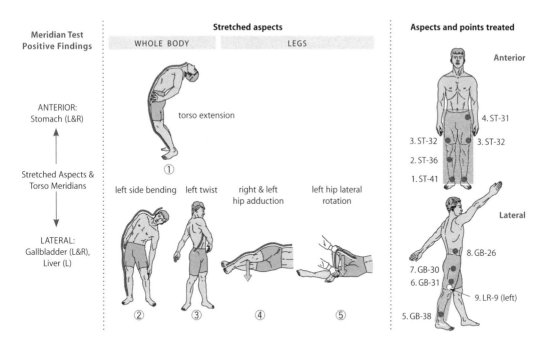

● **Figure IV–18**   Case study: 23-year-old rugby player

Observations

In the case of this rugby player in the back position, fatigue accumulated in the muscles on the medial and lateral aspects of his leg because he repeatedly practiced for a game with his opponent in mind. Furthermore, when this player hit (ran into his opponents with the ball), he twisted his upper body to the left, so it is likely that the lateral aspect of his low back was strained as well. This was clearly indicated as restrictions in M-Test movements of the lateral aspect.

As shown in Figure IV–19, the player feints to evade his opponent and moves abruptly in order to catch him off guard. This mainly takes the form of quick movements to either side. When a player constantly moves fast and abruptly changes direction or quickly stops, this causes fatigue, especially in the medial and lateral aspects of the legs. In the case of this player in the back position, it appears that the pain resulted from repeated stresses on the low back, which was affected by the fatigue in his legs.

In general, backs in rugby tend to accumulate fatigue in the low back, hamstrings, knees and ankles, which are stressed by running. Among these places, injuries tend to occur most often in the low back and hamstrings. When the M-Test is performed on injured backs, pain or restriction is often present with adduction, abduction, and flexion of the hip.

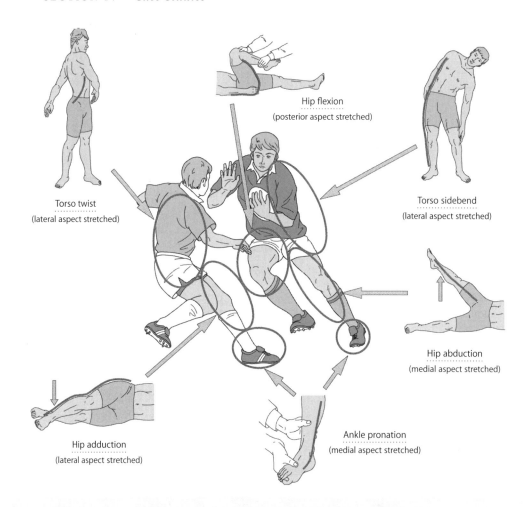

Hip flexion
(posterior aspect stretched)

Torso twist
(lateral aspect stretched)

Torso sidebend
(lateral aspect stretched)

Hip abduction
(medial aspect stretched)

Hip adduction
(lateral aspect stretched)

Ankle pronation
(medial aspect stretched)

In rugby, extension of the lateral aspect is most frequent in both offense and defense. Muscles in the lateral aspect become fatigued when movements like this are repeated over and over. This creates an imbalance in the body and this affects not only the legs, but the low back as well. Performing the M-Test allows one to identify the fatigued areas using simple movements.

● **Figure IV-19**   M-Test of movements involved in a feint

On the other hand, forwards tend to strain their necks and shoulders in scrums and tackles, as well as their lower back and legs from running. When the M-Test is performed on injured forwards, pain or restriction is often present with anterior flexion of the neck and torso, as well as flexion of the hip and dorsiflexion of the ankle.

Finally, the M-Test is highly effective for treating athletes because the test movements relate closely to how they use their bodies. Also, the M-Test can be used to prevent injuries, especially since the state of muscle fatigue is reflected in the outcome. In a sport like rugby, however, there are cases with structural damage. Therefore, if there is no effect with treatments based on the M-Test, it is important to have the injury examined by an orthopedic physician and not to delay medical treatment where necessary.

F. Kendo (fencing)

by Sawazaki Kenta

In the Japanese sport of Kendo, or fencing, simply hitting an opponent is not enough to score a point. The strike must be executed firmly with proper attitude and posture. In other words, there must be balance and coordination in the chain of movement from the legs and torso to the arms. In the attack, the Kendo player must stamp the floor with his front right foot as he strikes. Also, the grip on the *shinai* (bamboo sword) and the movement of the wrist must be correct to be able to swing the *shinai* smoothly. Thus the fine coordination of movements in the whole body, from the fingertips to the arms and legs and torso, is essential for success. Here I will present a case of neck pain originating from striking movements of Kendo, which was evaluated and treated using the M-Test.

● CASE STUDY: KENDO PLAYER WITH NECK PAIN

24-year-old male (student Kendo club coach)

CHIEF COMPLAINT: neck pain

HISTORY: Severe neck pain began the night before I saw him, and he had difficulty getting to sleep. He also felt nauseous. The pain was especially aggravated when he extended his neck. He had retired from competition himself, but was preparing his team for competition and so had pushed himself for three days in a row coaching and demonstrating.

M-Test positive findings (see M-Test Chart, p. 204)

ANTERIOR: 1 right & left (extension of neck)
 4 right & left (extension of shoulder)
 16 right (extension of hip)
 27 (extension of torso)

POSTERIOR: 2 left (flexion of neck)
 6 left (flexion of arm)
 18 left (flexion of hip)

LATERAL: None

Assessment & Treatment

1: right & left Lung meridian (LU-9)

4: right & left Large Intestine meridian (LI-11)

2: left Heart meridian (HT-7)

6: left Small Intestine meridian (SI-8)

16: right Stomach meridian (ST-36, 41)

18: left Kidney meridian (KI-7)

27: Stomach meridian Front *mu* point (CV-12)

Intradermal needles (Seirin press tacks) were retained in the above
  points.

Results

The neck pain was alleviated immediately after the treatment, and was
completely gone by the next day. The patient reported that the nausea
had also disappeared and he had slept well that night.

Observations

In the attacking movement of Kendo, it is said that about ten times
the body weight comes onto the forward foot that stamps down (Fig.
IV–20). So there is a big impact on the base of the toes (ball) of the
right foot, and there is a stress on the anterior right leg (right Stomach
meridian) to stop the body from going further forward (Fig. IV–22).
Also, the left leg, which must keep up with the forward movement
and support the body from behind by lifting the heel, is also stressed
in the posterior aspect (left Kidney meridian).

As far as the arms are concerned, the grip of the little finger of
the left hand is kept tight as the bamboo sword is raised (Fig. IV–21),
and the grip is tightened further as the sword is brought down (Fig. IV
–23). Thus the posterior aspect of the left arm is stressed (left Heart
meridian and left Small Intestine meridian). Also, to swing the sword
down, the grip is tightened by tensing the inside of the hands (Fig.
IV–24) and this stresses the anterior aspect of both arms (right and
left Lung meridian and right and left Large Intestine meridian).

The movements in Kendo are repetitive in nature, and it seems
that the neck pain occurred because muscles in the stressed aspects
became fatigued and the body got out of balance. Also, this Kendo
player was short and tends to extend his torso (posterior flexion)
when up against a taller opponent, especially when striking the face or
during a pushing match. This is probably related to the strain noted in
the anterior aspect of the body (1, 4, 16, and 27: Lung, Large Intestine,
and Stomach meridians).

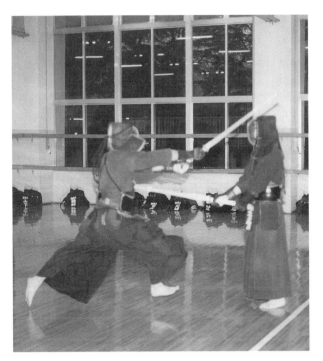

● **Figure IV–20**
Striking movement

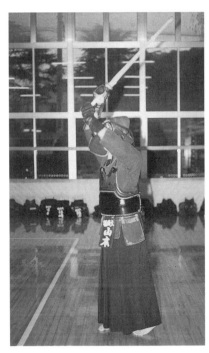

● **Figure IV–21**
Movement raising the bamboo sword

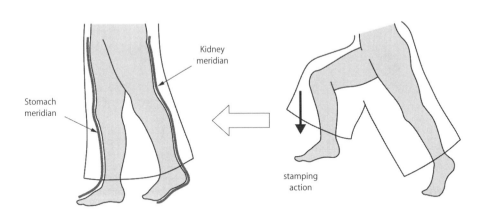

● **Figure IV–22**   Stress on the Stomach and Kidney meridians

By giving treatment based on the M-Test, I could also analyze the physical balance during the striking movement of Kendo. By performing acupuncture to adjust the body's balance, these treatments can be used for conditioning as well as injury prevention, and improved performance can be expected.

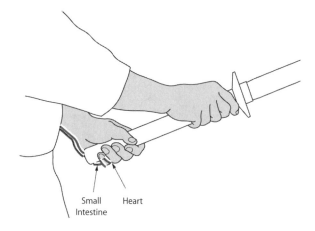

● **Figure IV–23**   Stress on the Heart and Small Intestine meridians

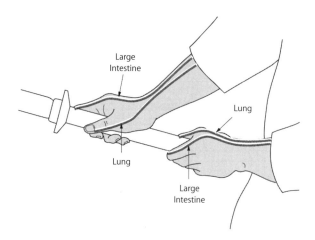

● **Figure IV–24**   Stress on the Lung and Large Intestine meridians

G. Tennis

by Yamashita Tomotaka

Tennis is a sport that is hard on the body, more so than it appears. During a match, a player must maintain a crouched position and keep the body weight over the medial aspect of the big toes; the knees must remain flexed. During the match, the knees are repeatedly extended and flexed. As for the arms, the dominant arm is used to grip the racket and hit the ball, so there is considerable stress on the shoulder and elbow. Furthermore, in all shots from the serve, stroke, volley, to the smash, whenever the ball is hit hard, one must step down hard, and all of the body weight comes down on the leg opposite the dominant arm. Thus strength in the legs is also required. Furthermore, during the serve when the ball overhead is hit hard, the torso that is initially extended goes into forward flexion in an instant. Thus strong abdominal muscles are also required. Here I will present a case of acupuncture treatment for a tennis player who had abdominal pain, which originated from serving.

● CASE STUDY: TENNIS PLAYER WITH ABDOMINAL PAIN

20-year-old male (student)

CHIEF COMPLAINT: pain in left abdomen

HISTORY: The pain began during a tournament in which he played in matches every day for over a week. He started feeling discomfort in his abdomen during one of the matches, and was no longer able to serve with a hundred percent of his strength. The abdominal pain was so bad after the last tennis match that he found it difficult to walk. He could no longer fully extend his torso (restriction in posterior flexion), so he came in the next day for acupuncture.

M-Test positive findings (see M-Test Chart, p. 204)

ANTERIOR: 16 left (extension of hip) prone
    17 left (flexion of knee) prone
    27 (extension of torso) standing

POSTERIOR: None

LATERAL: None

Assessment & Treatment

16 & 17: left Spleen meridian (SP-5, SP-6, SP-8), left Stomach meridian (ST-36, ST-41)

27: left Stomach meridian (ST-25, CV-12)

Intradermal needles (Seirin press tacks) were retained in the above points.

Although in this case there were abnormal findings only in the legs and torso, five-phase point combinations can be used to good effect when there are abnormal findings in the upper body and arms as well. By using five-phase combinations, meridians of the contralateral arm are treated along with meridians on the affected leg. The combinations I use most often are as follows:

ST-41, TB-10, SI-8: (earth, fire, and fire)

SP-5, LU-9: (earth and metal)

SP-2, PC-7, HT-7: (earth, fire, and fire)

ST-45, LI-11: (earth and metal)

Results

The patient could walk after the treatment, and the abdominal pain that he experienced when he served disappeared. He was able to play in his match the next day.

Observations

To serve in tennis, the knees are flexed (Fig. IV–25) and then the torso is extended (Fig. IV–26). In the case of a right-handed player, all the weight of the body comes onto the left leg (Fig. IV–27). Thus almost all the weight of the body comes over the medial aspect of the left big toe. This was the case for the player here, and there was a considerable strain on the Spleen and Stomach meridians of the left leg due to playing matches every day for over a week.

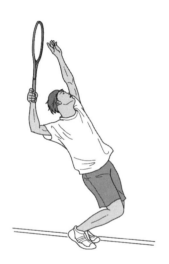

● **Figure IV–25**
Knees flexed

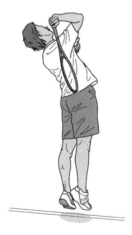

● **Figure IV– 26**
Torso extended

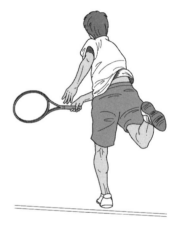

● **Figure IV–27**   Weight of whole body supported on one leg

Furthermore, in all shots from the serve, stroke, volley, to the smash, the shot is only effective when the knees are flexed deeply and the player steps into the shot with great force. Thus fatigue accumulates in the legs, and many players complain of problems in their anterior legs (especially with extension of the hip in the prone position, or movement 16 of the M-Test). Also, many players develop corns on the medial aspect of the big toes, and it's quite obvious that the Spleen meridian is repeatedly stressed.

The above case was abdominal pain originating from fatigue in the anterior legs, but performing acupuncture to relieve the fatigue in the legs often resolves other symptoms, regardless of whether it is pain in the shoulder, elbow, low back, or knee. Another thing I often experience in treating tennis players is that treating the leg opposite the dominant arm improves the symptom in the dominant arm (shoulder pain, elbow pain, etc.). This indicates that tennis is a sport that puts a strain especially on the dominant arm and the opposite leg (if a player is right-handed, the right arm and the left leg). Thus many problems in tennis players are a result of imbalances in the body caused by this contralateral stress.

The basic feature of tennis shot form is that the racket is swung with the dominant arm and the weight is placed on the opposite leg. Good results can be obtained when five-phase point combinations are used that take this feature into account, as well as treating contralateral points on the arms and legs. Also, as in this case, just relieving the fatigue in the legs based on the findings of the M-Test can prevent injuries and lead to better perfomance.

H. Swimming

by Matsumoto Miyuki

Most injuries in swimmers are a result of a comparatively small external force coming to bear repeatedly on the body. This is the so-called 'repetitive stress syndrome.' Although it varies depending on whether it is during the swimming season, a competitive swimmer must swim between 5,000 and 20,000 meters a day, and at least 40,000 meters a week. In some cases a swimmer will swim upwards of 70,000 meters a week. If this is done in a 25-meter pool, it amounts to 200 to 800 laps a day. The number of stokes per minute in the freestyle varies from swimmer to swimmer, but at maximum speed it is between 40 and 60 strokes a minute. In terms of the number of kicks, it is about the same number, between two and six beats per stoke. It is obvious from this perspective how the repetitive minor stress of a stroke (and kick) is compounded to cause considerable strain on the body.

Common injuries among swimmers include shoulder problems (impingement syndrome, subacromial bursitis, tendonitis of biceps brachii, rotator cuff damage, looseness and subluxation in acromioclavicular joint) and lumbar problems (myofascial low back pain, intervertebral disk herniation, and spondylolysis). This is followed by knee problems (medial collateral ligament damage, anterior patellar bursitis, and iliotibital ligament syndrome) among competitive breaststroke swimmers.

Also, even though it may be less common, we cannot overlook ankle pain from hyperextension (plantar flexion). Many swimmers

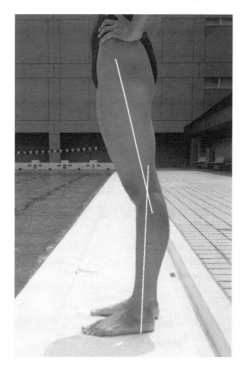

● **Figure IV-28**

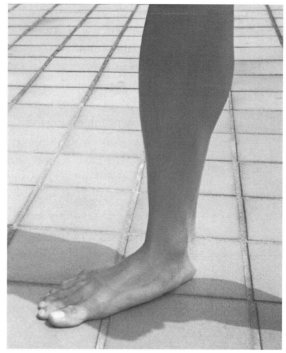

● **Figure IV-29**

have several structural anomalies such as hyper-extended knees (Fig. IV–28) and flat feet (Fig. IV–29), as well as knock-knee (genu valgum), bow leg (genu varum), and hyper-extension in elbows. Caution is necessary because swimmers with structural anomalies are prone to injury when running or doing weight training. Here I will present some approaches to treatment of injuries from swimming by using the M-Test to analyze the strain from various swimming styles.

1) Backstroke

The backstroke may appear to be a specialized from of swimming, but it has many features in common with freestyle swimming such as the rolling motion and six kicks per arm stroke. Also, backstroke swimmers tend to present similar findings as freestyle swimmers in the M-Test assessment. Because the backstroke swimmer faces up, however, there is a difference in that the abdominal muscles are used to maintain form. Another difference in the backstroke is that the rolling motion has to be greater than in the freestyle, or one cannot grab water. Furthermore, the kicking that is done with this large rolling motion of the body is performed with the leg twisted, so the kick is at a diagonal.

● CASE No. 1: SWIMMER WITH BACK PAIN

21-year-old female student (backstroke swimmer)

CHIEF COMPLAINT: low back pain (around the spine)

HISTORY: The pain in her low back became constant after returning from training camp. It was worse when she did turns and Pasalo kicks. Her total practice distance is under 10,000 meters a day.

M-Test positive findings (see M-Test Chart, p. 204)

ANTERIOR: right and left 27 (extension of torso)

POSTERIOR: 28 (flexion of torso)

LATERAL: 30 (twisting of torso)

Assessment & Treatment

28: Bladder meridian (BL-40, BL-36, BL-25)

27: Stomach meridian (ST-25 and ST-45 – LI-11 five-phase combination)

30: Girdle vessel (GB-26)

For treatment, needles were inserted into the above points and withdrawn immediately (simple insertion). During swimming practice, intradermal needles (Seirin press tacks) were retained in ST-25 and BL-25.

Results

The pain with movement was alleviated right after treatment, but the same pain returned after practice. Thus stretching, focusing on the anterior and posterior aspects, was suggested, and this daily self-care brought a gradual reduction in pain. The low back pain thereby diminished to just some fatigue and heaviness in the area when fatigue accumulated.

Observation

The back pain of this swimmer was at its worst when she bent forward, and was aggravated in the turns that require extreme flexion and also with the Pasalo kicks that involve both flexion and extension. Also, in the kicking motions of the backstroke, unlike other styles of swimming, effort is put into kicking down (hip extension) as much as kicking up. The hip joint has more power in flexion than it does in extension, but in the backstroke, the downward kick is achieved by hip extension. So, unlike other styles, the gluteus and hamstrings must be engaged more for a powerful kicking stroke; this puts more stress on the muscles in the posterior aspect. Also, this swimmer had hyper-extended knees, which stressed the posterior aspect of her knees during the downward kick. This is why treatment of the posterior aspect, including points like BL-40 and BL-36, was important.

Figure IV–30 is a photo showing this swimmer's form. It shows how the rolling motion of the body in the backstroke is greater than in freestyle, and also how the adduction of the shoulder is important. This swimmer had a beautiful rolling technique, but this made her twist her body back and forth with every stroke, which stretched and put tension on the Girdle vessel. Also, with the rolling motion and the twisting of her body, her kicks are seldom straight, and four out of six are done at a diagonal. As a result, backstroke swimmers tend to have abnormal findings with twisting motions. As far as findings in the anterior aspect, the stress from kicking seems to cause abnormalities in the anterior aspect, just as with freestyle swimmers (see next case.)

Unless the backstoke swimmer has a deep rolling technique, the line between the shoulder and the elbow is at a wide angle from that connecting the two shoulders, as shown in Figure IV–31. This stresses the shoulder and leads to shoulder pain, impingement syndrome, and other problems. Swimmers like the one shown in Figure IV–30, where the arm is pretty much in line with the shoulders, don't have that much shoulder pain. Aside from this 'catch-pull' motion of the backstroke, the recovery motion in the freestyle and butterfly can lead to impingement syndrome. These motions repeated over and over stress the anterior aspect of the arms, and the M-Test confirms how abnormalities tend to appear primarily in medial rotation of the shoulder with the elbow flexed. When this abnormality appears, stimulation of the Large Intestine meridian points (e.g., LI-5 or LI-11) is effective, except in acute and sub-acute stages.

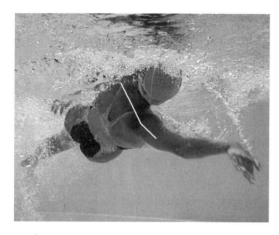

● **Figure IV–30**

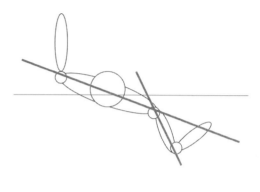

● **Figure IV–31**

IV

2) Freestyle

Unlike other styles of swimming, freestyle ('crawl') swimmers tend to do all their practice, from warm-up to cool-down, by swimming freestyle. This means that their bodies are under the same stresses at every stage of their practice. Thus imbalances tend to develop in the muscles of freestyle swimmers, and weak parts are even more susceptible to strain. Also, since swimmers of other styles do quite a bit of practice in the freestyle to strengthen heart function, one sometimes finds abnormalities common to freestyle swimmers in swimmers of other styles.

● CASE NO. 2: SWIMMER WITH SHOULDER AND BACK PAIN

22-year-old male student (long-distance swimmer)

CHIEF COMPLAINT: low back pain and left shoulder pain

HISTORY: He had been swimming long distances every day (over 15,000 meters) in preparation for the All-Japan Swimming Championship. He experienced low back pain when maintaining a streamlined posture under the water just after starting or during the turns. Also, he had low back pain and left shoulder pain during the reaching movement of the left arm.

M-Test positive findings (see M-Test Chart, p. 204)

ANTERIOR: 27 (extension of torso)

POSTERIOR: 6 left (flexion of shoulder)

LATERAL: 29 (lateral flexion of torso), 30 right (twisting of torso), 21 (adduction of hip)

Treatment

Filliform needles were inserted but not retained as follows: ST-25, ST-45, and LI-11 (five-phase combination) for movement 27; GB-26 (Girdle vessel) for movements 29 and 30. With this, the pain associated with movement 21 was alleviated, as well as the pain associated with movements 27, 29, and 30. To consolidate the effects, GB-31 (Gall-bladder meridian) was treated for movement 21, and HT-7 and SP-2 (five-phase combination) on the left were treated for movement 6.

Results

The pain with movement was almost completely resolved after treatment, but a similar pain returned after practice. As treatments continued, however, the number of movements that were positive after practice declined. Nevertheless, the occurrence of pain with movements 27 and 30 (left) continued.

Observation

In the sport of swimming, movements are generally symmetrical, but the reason this swimmer developed a difference in the same right and left movements is probably because he was using an irregular kick, which is seen in long-distance swimmers who use a four-beat kick. He maintained his rhythm, balance, and timing during one stroke with a strong downward kick of the left leg as the right arm entered the water, as shown in Figure IV–32. He did not maintain his balance with the opposite left arm / right leg stroke, as shown in Figure IV–33-1. He maintained his balance by reaching his right leg slightly out to the side and also by reaching his pronated left arm out to the side, as shown in Figure IV–33-2. In addition, he is a right-side breather, which probably added to the stress in his left shoulder and caused the shoulder and low back pain.

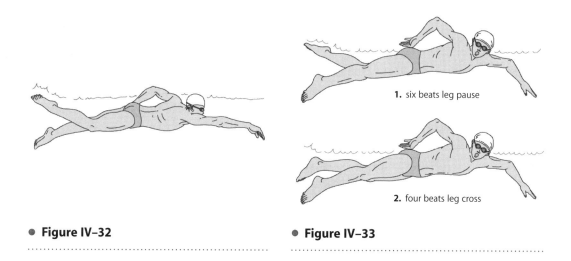

1. six beats leg pause

2. four beats leg cross

● **Figure IV–32**

● **Figure IV–33**

Analyzing his characteristic right arm / left leg stroke with the M-Test, the arm is stretched on the anterior aspect in pronation and the trunk and legs are also stretched on the anterior aspect with the hyper-dorsiflexion of the left ankle. The pain was instantly reduced when I treated ST-45 (a point on the meridian distal to the stressed ankle joint) along with the five-phase combination point LI-11.

Also, I decided it was important to treat the anterior trunk because this swimmer was aware that he also experienced low back pain when he was fatigued and slouched into a posture of excessive kyphosis. Therefore I also treated ST-25, and the low back pain was almost completely alleviated. As for the problem in his left shoulder joint, since its flexion movement was abnormal with the M-Test, I treated HT-7 along with SP-2.

Nevertheless, abnormal M-Test findings continued to appear with extension and twisting of the torso after swimming practice. These are abnormal findings that commonly appear in competitive backstroke and freestyle swimmers. Swimmers use a rolling motion of the shoulder to extend their stroke further in the freestyle, just as they do in the backstroke. In addition to extending their arm overhead as it enters the water, they medially rotate the shoulder to reach as far forward in the water as they can. The upper body tips in the direction of the reaching arm in this movement, so the swimmer must balance this with his legs. Just as in walking, where balance is maintained by twisting the body by swinging the right arm forward as the left leg takes a step, in swimming, the left leg is kicked downward powerfully as the right arm enters the water (Fig. IV–32).

The pain caused by this movement can be reproduced by the twisting motion of the torso (30) in the M-Test. This is also a common finding among backstroke swimmers. Furthermore, not just freestyle swimmers, but backstroke and butterfly swimmers as well have great flexibility in their ankles, which easily exceeds the normal 45 degrees of dosiflexion. Two-to-six leg beats per stroke are used in the freestyle, six leg beats are used in the backstroke, and two beats are used in the butterfly. Thus the anterior aspect of the legs (Stomach meridian) is stretched most frequently and this shows up as an abnormal finding of extension of the torso (stretching anterior aspect of legs) (Fig. IV–34).

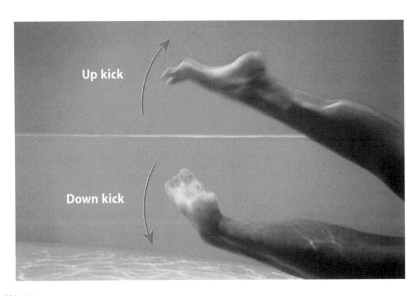

● **Figure IV–34**

Also, among freestyle swimmers there are those who complain of pain in their rotator cuff when swimming all out. This is probably caused by a reduction in blood flow to the supraspinatus muscle with the internal rotation and adduction movements of the shoulder. In the M-Test, this problem often appears as abnormal findings in horizontal extension (movement 8) of the shoulder or medial rotation of the arm (pronation, movement 5). These findings indicate that the anterior aspect (Large Intestine meridian) is under the greatest stress, so the anterior aspect of the arm (usually LI-11) is treated for best results.

3) Breaststroke

Among the four competitive swimming styles, the breaststroke is the only one in which the propulsion from the legs is greater than that from the arms. In freestyle, the arms account for 60 to 70 percent of the forward momentum, in the backstroke about 60 percent, and in the butterfly 50 percent. By contrast, the arms account for only about 40 percent of the forward momentum in the breaststroke. Thus in this event, in which leg strength means so much, flexibility of the leg is essential, especially in the ankles and knees. Nevertheless, the hyper-flexibility or misalignment of these joints often leads to instability in the joint and becomes the cause of injuries. There is even a characteristic problem called 'breaststroke knee,' which is primarily an abnormality in the medial collateral ligament. Also, one must be careful because there tends to be more flat feet with fallen arches (Fig. IV–29) among breaststroke swimmers than among swimmers of other styles.

● CASE NO. 3: SWIMMER WITH KNEE PAIN

20-year-old female student (breaststroke swimmer)

CHIEF COMPLAINT: left knee pain

HISTORY: She has had this pain since her high school days, which is elicited when kicking out from the position of knee flexion. She has been swimming about 10,000 meters a day.

M-Test positive findings (see M-Test Chart, p. 204)

ANTERIOR: 27 (extension of torso), 17 left (knee flexion)

POSTERIOR: None

LATERAL: None

Treatment

Needles were inserted but not retained in SP-5 and LU-9 on the left for movement 17, and in ST-25 bilaterally for movement 27. Also, intradermal (press tack) needles were placed in these points during her swimming practice.

Results

The pain with movement almost disappeared after the first treatment, but the pain returned after practice, so I gave her instructions on how to do self-massage and stretch, primarily for the Spleen meridian. We also continued weekly treatments and the knee pain gradually subsided.

Observations

In the breaststroke, either the wave-stroke or the flat-stroke is used. The wave-stroke is a technique that includes elements of the butterfly. It makes use of the rocking motion in the upper body to ride over the water, as if riding a wave. Currently, the wave-stroke is the mainstream technique in the breaststroke. The flat-stroke is the opposite in that the up-and-down movement of the body is limited and resistance is kept to a minimum by staying close to the surface of the water. There are also two kicking techniques in the breaststroke. One is the whip kick where the knees are kept closer together while the heels are drawn back to the hips (Fig.IV–35a). The other is the wedge kick where the knees are spread wide apart like a frog and the heels are drawn back to the hips (Fig.IV–35b). Currently, the whip kick is the mainstream kicking technique in the breaststroke. This technique

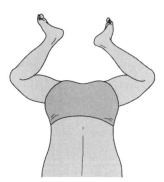

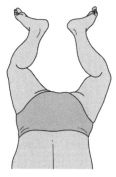

The common breaststroke form: The knees are wide apart (slightly over shoulder width) when flexed and the heels are pulled up close to the hips. The legs are kicked out diagonally and the knees can be extended strongly and fully each time in this movement.

An advanced breaststroke form: The knees are kept closer together when flexed and the feet are not brought as close to the hips. The ankles are kept loose and the toes are pointed outward so that water is captured more with the ankles than the legs during the kick.

● **Figure IV–35a** Wedge kick

● **Figure IV–35b** Whip kick

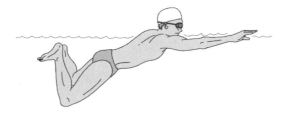

● **Figure IV–36**

increases the stress on the medial aspect of the knee joint and tends to cause knee pain.

This swimmer also swam with the wave-stroke whip kick combination, and complained of knee pain when she began to kick from the position with the heels close to the hips (knee flexion, ankle dosiflexion, and pronation) (Fig. IV–36). It seems that breaststroke swimmers often complain of pain during this movement. This is a movement that utilizes the flexibility of the knees and ankles to the utmost, and it seems to stretch the Spleen meridian to the utmost with the pronation of the ankle. Strain in this aspect was reflected in the M-Test, and also abnormality was detected in knee flexion, which stretches the Spleen and Stomach meridians. The knee pain was immediately alleviated when SP-5 (on the aspect that is stretched) was needled along with LU-9. Also, the style of this swimmer was to arch her torso on the surface of the water to create more of a wave, and this probably placed excessive stress on her anterior torso. I therefore also treated ST-25. This reduced the low back pain that she had been experiencing from time to time.

I often use points on the Spleen or Liver meridian for knee pain in breaststroke swimmers. In this case, there were no abnormalities in movements involving the Liver meridian, but when abduction of the hip or the Patrick's test is positive, I recommend treating the Liver meridian. I usually use the LV-8 and KI-1 five-phase combination. I also use this combination for swimmers with flat feet.

With the M-Test, treatment is given after confirming the movements that cause pain, so one works with an awareness of movements associated with the pain. This makes this a treatment system with a high rate of reproducibility. Swimming is sport in the water, and furthermore, swimmers tend to be very flexible, so sometimes it is difficult to reproduce the pain out of the pool. Likewise it is often hard to discriminate restrictions in the movements of swimmers with the M-Test because they are very flexible. In such cases, along with careful questioning, one must visualize the anatomy of the area with pain, and deduce the meridians that are strained and treat the affected area accordingly.

I. Volleyball

by Fukazawa Hiroki

In volleyball there are various roles for players including receiver, setter, and attacker. Regardless of the position, however, all players must stay in a forward-leaning posture of readiness so as to be able to move quickly in any direction — forward, backward, right, left, up, or down. From this posture they have to jump, or attack, and stop and go repeatedly in order to receive or hit the ball again and again. This vigorous shifting of weight back and forth puts a great stress on the body and the anterior legs. Especially the anterior thighs tend to become fatigued. Here I will present a case of leg pain originating from intensive volleyball practice that was analyzed and treated using the M-Test.

● CASE STUDY: VOLLEYBALL PLAYER WITH LEG PAIN

18-year-old female (student with a sports scholarship)

CHIEF COMPLAINT: Pain in the front of both legs

HISTORY: The pain began during practice and was hard to bear. It seemed like the soreness in the muscles became aggravated. She had a difficult time braking with stop-and-go movements. Now she is unable to jump or even remain in the forward-leaning posture.

M-Test positive findings (see M-Test Chart, p. 204)

ANTERIOR: 16 right and left, 17 right and left, 27

POSTERIOR: 18 right and left

LATERAL: 20 right, 21 right and left

Assessment & Treatment

ANTERIOR: 16 right and left, 17 right and left, 27: Spleen and Stomach meridian on both sides
  (SP-10, ST-36, ST-34, ST-32)

POSTERIOR: 18 right and left: Kidney meridian on both sides

Five-phase combination of water and wood points (KI-1 and LR-8)

LATERAL: 20 right: Liver meridian on right

Five-phase combination of wood and fire points (LR-2, PC-9, and HT-9)

21 right and left: Gallbladder meridian on both sides (GB-38)

Seirin red (0.16mm) 30mm needles were inserted just a few millimeters in each of the above points; the needles were not retained.

Results

The pain was alleviated after the treatment and she said that her legs felt lighter and that it was easier to walk. Her complaint was completely resolved with another treatment two days later.

Observations

This patient had just entered college from a high school that frequently made the Inter High School Meet volleyball championships. She told me that the amount of practice in college was far greater than what she was used to in high school. The day she felt the pain, in addition to the regular practice, she had practiced jumping and barbell squats. Obviously, this excessive amount of practice was something her body could not tolerate. The leg pain apparently came from extreme muscle fatigue. This was a case of 'overuse syndrome.'

The basic posture of receiving a ball, in which a player bends forward (Figs. IV–37 & 38), puts stress on the Spleen and Stomach meridians on the anterior aspect. This pattern of stress is the same while jumping, landing, and moving around in a crouched position. This is why treating points on the Spleen and Stomach meridians brought remarkable results. This is a relatively simple case where the patient's complaint and the positive findings of the M-Test matched. When excessive fatigue causes restrictions in stretching a certain aspect (meridian), it seems that the aspect that is strained can be treated directly, and that treatment can be started from the local area.

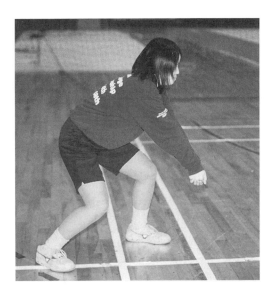

● **Figure IV–37**

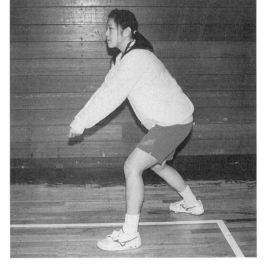

● **Figure IV–38**

J. Golf

by Sakuraba Hinata

I will briefly discuss the injuries that develop from the golf swing and how to prevent them, and examine the relationship between the golf swing and the meridians. Finally, I will present a case study and an interesting and clinically useful result obtained from my recent studies.

In order to generate speed and power in a golf swing, one must use the spine as an axis and skillfully employ the legs and hip joint to make a large swing using the shoulder girdle. Naturally, injuries tend to occur in these muscles (in the lumbar area especially on the right, in the upper back, as well as in the neck and shoulder). The primary cause of injuries is overuse. Alternative medicine like massage, acupuncture, and chiropractic are often used to treat such injuries. To prevent injury it is important for the golfer to swing the club in a way that is suited to his body and does not cause undue strain. Also, he must constantly monitor his own condition and be quick to notice any change due to stress or mental and physical fatigue. It is important to resolve these issues as quickly as possible with self-care and appropriate medical care. The therapist must apply M-Tests with some understanding of golf and must advise the golfer on appropriate self-care, including stretching and strengthening, in addition to the treatment.

The golf swing can be divided into several stages: take-back, back swing, top swing, bottom swing, impact, follow-through, and finish. From the bottom swing to the impact, the torso undergoes a right side bend and a twist to the left (Fig. IV–39). Activity in the back and gluteal muscles intensifies at this moment. Injuries in the right lumbar area tend to occur from this movement. Examining the relationship to the meridians, the Gallbladder meridian is stretched in the left leg, the Stomach meridian is stretched in the right leg, and both the lateral meridians (Liver and Gallbladder) are stretched in the torso. In the clinic, I often see restrictions in the left hip joint, notably movement 20 (external rotation of hip) and movement 21 (adduction of hip). Thus the treatment must target restrictions in the left hip joint. Also, the arms must be examined with the M-Test movements specific to the shoulder, elbow, and wrist joints to determine which meridians are affected.

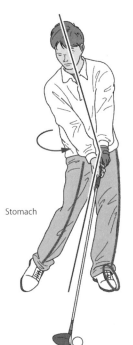

Stomach   Gallbladder

● **Figure IV–39**
Relationship between impact and meridians

- CASE STUDY: GOLFER WITH DISCOMFORT IN NECK

35-year-old male (employee at a driving range)

GOLFING HISTORY: 18 years, average score 74, best score 64

EVALUATION METHOD: He hit 100 balls toward a target 150 yards away (using a 7 iron) and then was given a treatment, after which he hit 50 more balls.

HISTORY: He had surgery on the left knee ten years ago for a meniscus tear. During rounds of golf he feels some heaviness in his left leg if he becomes tired, but usually it is not a problem.

CURRENT CONDITION: He has some discomfort in the neck due to some neck strain while sleeping about a week ago. He also feels minor restriction in movement of his left leg. Otherwise he has no problems and he is healthy mentally and physically.

M-Test positive findings (see M-Test Chart, p. 204)

ANTERIOR: None

POSTERIOR: 2 (neck flexion), 18 left (hip flexion), 19 left (hip flexion with knee in flexion)

LATERAL: 20 left (Patrick's test)

Treatment

Intradermal needles (Seirin pyonex) were placed in each the points. The discomfort in the neck resolved with left HT-7 and left SI-5 (Heart and Small Intestine meridians). The lateral meridians (Liver and Gallbladder) or the anterior meridians (Spleen and Stomach) were indicated by the M-Test and the above analysis of the swing movement, but treatment of the Kidney and Bladder (especially BL-65) was the most effective. According to five-phase theory, the Kidney and Bladder (water) meridians are in a controlling relationship with the Heart and Small Intestine (fire) meridians. It seems that the fifth metatarsal bone where BL-65 is located receives the weight of the body during the impact and follow-through phase of the swing, so it was probably strained.

Results

He started to complain of fatigue since he wasn't used to hitting that many balls in practice, but he commented that his overall balance was better. The intradermal needles that were taped on caused almost no sensation while he hit the balls.

Observations

In any sport the sense of being balanced is very important. This case

IV

deviated somewhat from the principle of treatment at first, but good results were obtained by treating the subject based on an analysis of his movements and correlating the restrictions with the meridians. Even though he experienced some fatigue, the subject was able to regain overall balance. Furthermore, by using the M-Test, which assesses the entire body for problematic movements, I was able to find problems in movement of which the subject was unaware. Golf is a continuous repetition of walking and swinging, and I see many cases where fatigue in the legs leads to low back pain. Assessing problems in the legs in advance with the M-Test is an effective way to prevent low back pain and other strains and injuries. Also, among golfers I often find restriction in pronation of the right forearm and adduction of the left hip. These restrictions have an adverse effect in the movement sequence of swinging the club. Assessing such problems in movement and providing the appropriate treatment can improve the golfer's performance.

K. Baton Twirling

by Suefuji Kumiko

Baton twirling as a competitive event is not just about twirling the baton with one's hands, but involves many different techniques, and some high level skills are required. Also, along with perfection of individual techniques, the overall balance of the performance, the timing with the music, and artistic expression are important elements. Therefore the smooth coordination of a series of movements and techniques and the balance of the entire body are indispensable. Nevertheless, in baton twirling the most frequent maneuver is to hold and twirl the baton in the right hand, so it cannot be denied that the stress is often greater on that side of the body. Among the baton twirlers who complain of low back pain, there are cases that can be attributed to the repeated strain on the upper body, especially the dominant arm. Here I will present a case where one-sided stress on the arm most likely caused low back pain.

● CASE STUDY: BATON TWIRLER WITH LOW BACK PAIN

15-year-old female (student)

CHIEF COMPLAINT: Pain in the low back

HISTORY: About two years ago she experienced low back pain while practicing baton twirling and went to see an orthopedic doctor. X-rays showed no abnormality and she was told it was due to "over-use." She returned weekly for instructions (unclear for how long) on rehab exercises, but the back pain persisted. She was planning to perform in a competition in just three weeks, and her back pain had become worse the more she practiced.

M-Test positive findings (see M-Test Chart, p. 204)

ANTERIOR: 16 right and left (hip extension), 27 (torso extension)

POSTERIOR: 28 (torso flexion)

LATERAL: 29 left (torso side bend)

Point Selection

① Five-phase points: bilateral ST-41, right TB-10 and SI-8 (combination of earth and fire), left KI-7 and right LU-5 (combination of metal and water)

② *Mu* and *shu* points: BL-13, BL-14, and BL-15 in the right interscapular area, BL-20, BL-21, BL-22, BL-23, and BL-26 in the left lumbar area (back *shu* points), and CV-12 (front *mu* point)

③ Tender points: right LU-1 and right SI-14 (the most tender point on medial border of scapula)

Treatment

First treatment: Seirin red (0.16mm) 40mm needles were inserted in the points in ① and ② but the needles were not retained. Next, intradermal needles (Seirin press tacks) were placed in TB-10 and SI-8 on the right arm and a tender point on the medial border of the right scapula. The low back pain was substantially reduced after this first treatment.

Second treatment (about 4 weeks later): 27 (torso extension) and 28 (torso flexion) were the only positive findings in the M-Test before the treatment. The back pain was especially aggravated by movements that stretched the anterior aspect (extension). So after treating the points in ① and ②, the patient was asked to perform movements 27 (torso extension) and 28 (torso flexion) while pressure was applied on the points in ③. In this way, it was confirmed that these points alleviated the back pain. Intradermal needles were placed in these two points and the low back pain was substantially reduced.

Observations

In the basic maneuver of baton twirling, the arm is held at the level of the shoulder with the elbow extended, and the baton is twirled with the pronation and supination of the wrist and fingers. Pronation especially involves the thumb and index fingers and stretches the Lung and Large Intestine meridians (Fig. IV–40). Supination, the reverse movement with the wrist and fingers, stretches the Heart and Small Intestine meridians (Fig. IV–41). As the stress of these movements builds up, the arm and shoulder girdle take on tension. From the

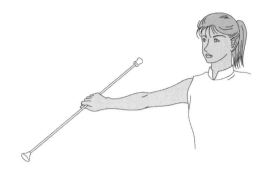

● **Figure IV–40** Pronation with wrist and fingers (Lung and Large Intestine meridians)

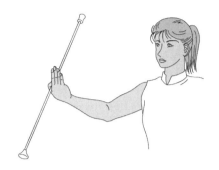

● **Figure IV–41** Supination (Heart and Small Intestine meridians)

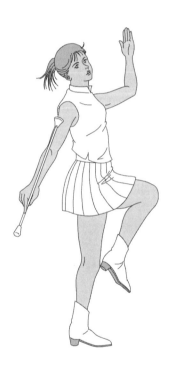

● **Figure IV–42** Extension of right arm (anterior meridians stretched)

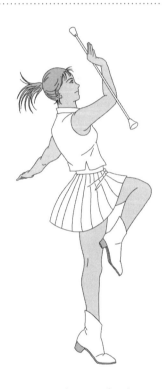

● **Figure IV–43** Flexion of right arm (posterior meridians stretched)

shoulder this stress is of course transmitted to the torso, but according to meridian theory, the stress also travels to the front *mu* and back *shu* points on each of the meridians associated with the anterior, posterior, and lateral aspects.

The patient in this case had begun to train seriously for competition from about the fourth grade, and stress had built up in her right elbow and shoulder for a long time. The fact that LU-1 and SI-14 on the right side were among the most effective points in the treatment indicates that the repeated extension of the right arm (stretching the anterior meridians; see Fig. IV–42) and flexion of the right arm (stretching the posterior meridians; see Fig. IV–43) had put stress on her shoulder girdle. This stress only increased with the intensified practice in preparation for competition. The stress probably exceeded her physical limits and her body went far enough out of balance to cause low back pain.

I deduced that the problem was in the upper body (especially the interscapular area) by questioning this patient about repetitive movements (identifying the strained meridians) and performing M-Tests to find abnormal movements. In the supine position she felt no discomfort with movement 18 (hip flexion) that extends the posterior leg, but she felt pain in the interscapular area and low back when she raised her upper body to get up. Also, she felt pain in these areas when straightening up from a forward bend in the standing position. This is how I arrived at the above-mentioned effective points of ③.

To restore the proper linkage and smooth movement of the body as a whole, and to achieve physical balance, the aspects that are stressed must be identified, along with restrictions or reduction in movement. The treatment must aim to reduce these imbalances. This approach, in addition to preventing injury, improves the conditioning of athletes and enhances their performance. I have presented a case in which I found an imbalance in the upper body by using the M-Test to identify the cause of low back pain. Acupuncture on points in the upper body substantially alleviated the low back pain.

....

Points Frequently Used in Sports Acupuncture

Points in Table Form

THIS IS A LIST of the primary points on the arm and leg as well as the front *mu* (Alarm) and back *shu* (Associated) points on the torso. Only 60 of the acupuncture points most useful for improving balance and movement for sports have been included. There are many possible point selections based on each practitioner's knowledge and experience, so there is no need to limit oneself to these points as long as the M-Test is used to assess movements. These tables have been configured so that one can easily identify which aspect and meridian each point is associated with.

ANTERIOR POINTS

Points on Arm (see Figs. 1 & 2)

Chinese Name	Japanese Name	Abbreviation	Meridian	No. in Figure
Taiyuan	Tai-en	LU-9	Lung	1
Chize	Shakutaku	LU-5	Lung	2
Jingqu	Keikyo	LU-8	Lung	3
Erjian	Jikan	LI-2	Large Intestine	4
Quchi	Kyokuchi	LI-11	Large Intestine	5
Shangyang	Shoyo	LI-1	Large Intestine	6

Points on Leg (see Figs. 3 & 4)

Chinese Name	Japanese Name	Abbreviation	Meridian	No. in Figure
Dadu	Daito	SP-2	Spleen	1
Shangqiu	Shokyu	SP-5	Spleen	2
Taibai	Taihaku	SP-3	Spleen	3
Lidui	Reida	ST-45	Stomach	4
Jiexi	Kaikei	ST-41	Stomach	5
Sanli	Sanli	ST-36	Stomach	6

POSTERIOR POINTS

Points on Arm (see Figs. 1 & 2)

Chinese Name	Japanese Name	Abbreviation	Meridian	No. in Figure
Shaochong	Shosho	HT-9	Heart	7
Shenmen	Shinmon	HT-7	Heart	8
Shaofu	Shofu	HT-8	Heart	9
Houxi	Koukei	SI-3	Small Intestine	10
Xiaohai	Shokai	SI-8	Small Intestine	11
Yanggu	Yokoku	SI-5	Small Intestine	12

POSTERIOR POINTS, CONT.

Points on Leg (see Figs. 3 & 4)

Chinese Name	Japanese Name	Abbreviation	Meridian	No. in Figure
Yongquan	Yusen	KI-1	Kidney	7
Fuliu	Fukuryu	KI-7	Kidney	8
Yingu	Inkoku	KI-10	Kidney	9
Zhiyin	Shi-in	BL-67	Bladder	10
Shugu	Sok-koku	BL-65	Bladder	11
Tonggu	Tsukoku	BL-66	Bladder	12

LATERAL POINTS

Points on Arm (see Figs. 1 & 2)

Chinese Name	Japanese Name	Abbreviation	Meridian	No. in Figure
Zhongchong	Chusho	PC-9	Pericardium	13
Daling	Dairyo	PC-7	Pericardium	14
Laogong	Rokyu	PC-8	Pericardium	15
Zhongzhu	Chusho	TB-3	Triple Burner	16
Tianjing	Tensei	TB-10	Triple Burner	17
Zhigou	Shiko	TB-6	Triple Burner	18

Points on Leg (see Figs. 3 & 4)

Chinese Name	Japanese Name	Abbreviation	Meridian	No. in Figure
Xingjian	Koukan	LR-2	Liver	13
Ququan	Kyokusen	LR-8	Liver	14
Dadun	Daiton	LR-1	Liver	15
Xiaxi	Kyokei	GB-43	Gallbladder	16
Yangfu	Yoho	GB-38	Gallbladder	17
Linqi	Rinkyu	GB-41	Gallbladder	18

TORSO POINTS

Front *mu* points (see Fig. 5)

● ANTERIOR POINTS

Chinese Name	Japanese Name	Abbreviation	Meridian/organ	No. in Figure
Zhongfu	Chufu	LU-1	Lung	1
Tianshu	Tensu	ST-25	Large Intestine	2
Zhangmen	Shomon	LR-13	Spleen	3
Zhongwan	Chukan	CV-12	Stomach	4

● POSTERIOR POINTS

Chinese Name	Japanese Name	Abbreviation	Meridian/organ	No. in Figure
Juque	Koketsu	CV-14	Heart	5
Guanyuan	Kangen	CV-4	Small Intestine	6
Jingmen	Keimon	GB-25	Kidney	7
Zhongji	Chukyoku	CV-3	Bladder	8

● LATERAL POINTS

Chinese Name	Japanese Name	Abbreviation	Meridian/organ	No. in Figure
Danzhong	Danchu	CV-17	Pericardium	9
Shimen	Sekimon	CV-5	Triple Burner	10
Qimen	Kimon	LR-14	Liver	11
Riyue	Jitsugetsu	GB-24	Gallbladder	12

TORSO POINTS, CONT.

Back *shu* points (see Fig. 6)

● ANTERIOR POINTS

Chinese Name	Japanese Name	Abbreviation	Meridian/organ	No. in Figure
Feishu	Haiyu	BL-13	Lung	1
Dachangshu	Daichoyu	BL-25	Large Intestine	2
Pishu	Hiyu	BL-20	Spleen	3
Weishu	Iyu	BL-21	Stomach	4

● POSTERIOR POINTS

Chinese Name	Japanese Name	Abbreviation	Meridian/organ	No. in Figure
Xinshu	Shinyu	BL-15	Heart	5
Xiaochangshu	Shochoyu	BL-27	Small Intestine	6
Shenshu	Jinyu	BL-23	Kidney	7
Pangguangshu	Bokoyu	BL-28	Bladder	8

● LATERAL POINTS

Chinese Name	Japanese Name	Abbreviation	Meridian/organ	No. in Figure
Jueyinshu	Ketsu-inyu	BL-14	Pericardium	9
Sanjiaoshu	Sanshoyu	BL-22	Triple burner	10
Ganshu	Kanyu	BL-18	Liver	11
Danshu	Tanyu	BL-19	Gallbladder	12

A

Main Acupuncture Points of the Arm (Fig. 1)

These illustrations show the location of the main acupuncture points on the hand and arm. The points associated with the anterior aspect are black, those associated with the posterior aspect are dark blue, and those associated with the lateral and medial aspects are light blue.

1 LU-9

3 LU-8

4 LI-2

6 LI-1

7 HT-9

8 HT-7

9 HT-8

13 PC-9

14 PC-7

15 PC-8

16 TB-2

18 TB-6

● anterior

● posterior

● lateral / medial

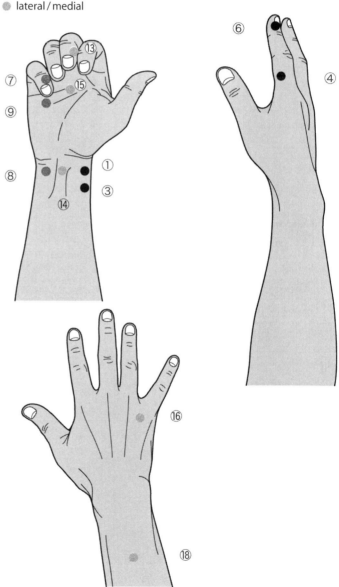

Main Acupuncture Points of the Arm (Fig. 2)

The acupuncture points on the anterior aspect are numbered from 1 to 6, those on the posterior aspect are numbered from 7 to 12, and those on the lateral or medial aspect are numbered from 13 to 18. Also the first three numbers in each group are yin meridian points and the last three numbers in each group are yang meridian points.

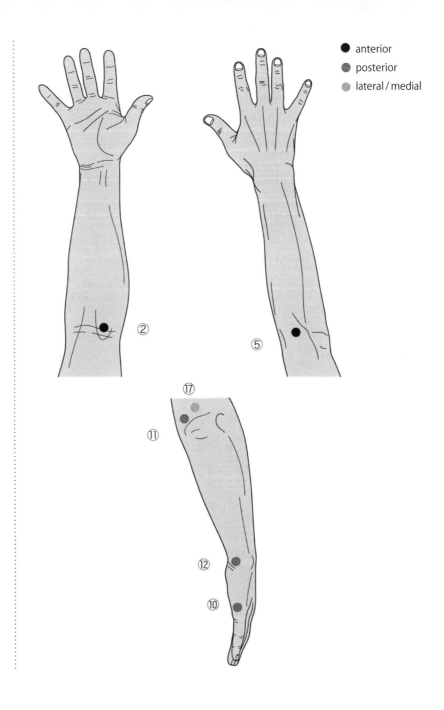

2	LU-5
5	LI-11
10	SI-3
11	SI-8
12	SI-5
17	TB-10

● anterior
● posterior
● lateral / medial

Main Acupuncture Points of the Leg (Fig. 3)

These illustrations show the location of the main acupuncture points on the foot and leg. The points associated with the anterior aspect are black, those associated with the posterior aspect are dark blue, and those associated with the lateral and medial aspects are light blue.

1   SP-2

2   SP-5

3   SP-3

4   ST-45

5   ST-41

7   KI-1

10 BL-67

11 BL-65

12 BL-66

13 LR-2

15 LR-1

16 GB-43

18 GB-41

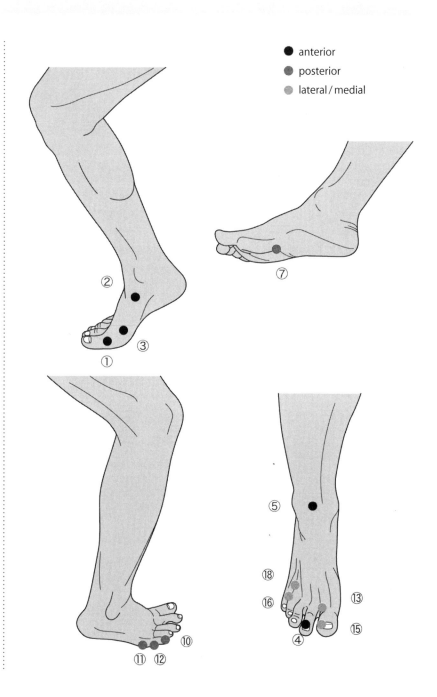

Main Acupuncture Points of the Leg (Fig. 4)

A

The acupuncture points on the anterior aspect are numbered from 1 to 6, those on the posterior aspect are numbered from 7 to 12, and those on the lateral or medial aspect are numbered from 13 to 18. Also the first three numbers in each group are yin meridian points and the last three numbers in each group are yang meridian points.

6   ST-36

8   KI-7

9   KI-10

14   LR-8

17   GB-38

● anterior
● posterior
● lateral / medial

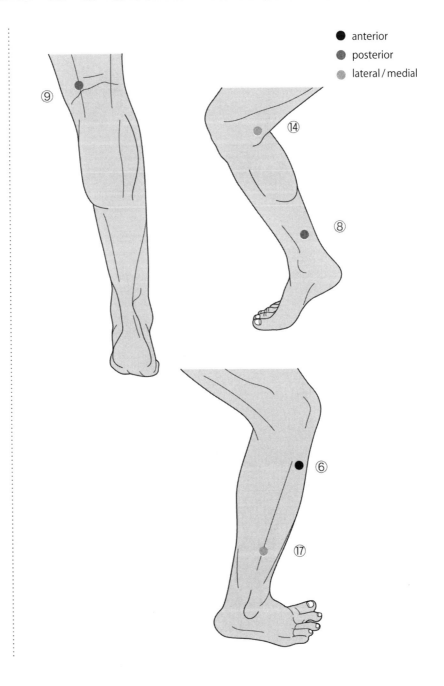

Main Acupuncture Points of the Torso (Fig. 5)

These illustrations show the location of the Alarm (*mu*) points of each meridian. The Alarm points are not always on the meridian with which they are associated, so the abbreviation of the meridian is shown in brackets after each point. Alarm points on the anterior aspect are numbered from 1 to 4, those on the posterior aspect are numbered from 5 to 8, and those on the lateral aspect are numbered from 9 to 12. The first two numbers in each group are points on the arm meridians, and the last two numbers in each group are points on the leg meridians. Among the numbers thus paired, the lesser number represents a yin meridian point, while the greater number represents a yang meridian point. Thus, for example, ① LU-1 is associated with the Lung meridian and ② ST-25 is associated with the Large Intestine meridian.

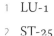

1	LU-1
2	ST-25
3	LR-13
4	CV-12
5	CV-14
6	CV-4
7	GB-25
8	CV-3
9	CV-17
10	CV-5
11	LR-14
12	GB-24

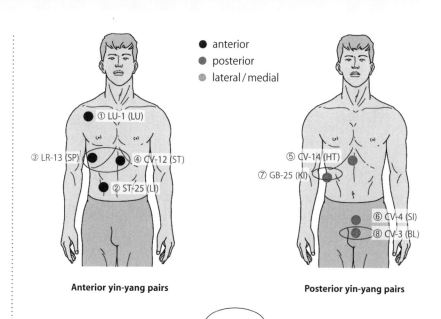

● anterior
● posterior
● lateral / medial

Anterior yin-yang pairs

Posterior yin-yang pairs

ALARM POINTS OF YIN-YANG PAIRS

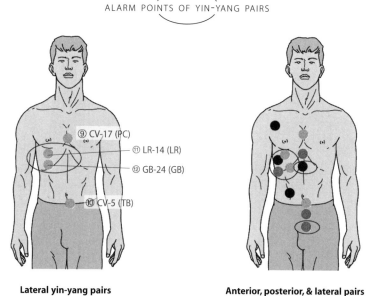

Lateral yin-yang pairs

Anterior, posterior, & lateral pairs

Main Acupuncture Points of the Torso (Fig. 6)

These illustrations show the location of the Associated (*shu*) points of each meridian. All the Associated points are located on the Bladder meridian. The abbreviation of the associated meridian is shown in brackets after each point. As in the previous figure, Associated points on the anterior aspect are numbered from 1 to 4, those on the posterior aspect are numbered from 5 to 8, and those on the lateral aspect are numbered from 9 to 12. The first two numbers in each group are points on the arm meridians, and the last two numbers in each group are points on the leg meridians. Among the numbers thus paired, the lesser number represents a yin meridian point, while the greater number represents a yang meridian point. Thus, for example, ① BL-13 is associated with the Lung meridian and ② BL-25 is associated with the Large Intestine meridian.

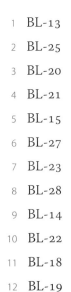

1   BL-13
2   BL-25
3   BL-20
4   BL-21
5   BL-15
6   BL-27
7   BL-23
8   BL-28
9   BL-14
10 BL-22
11 BL-18
12 BL-19

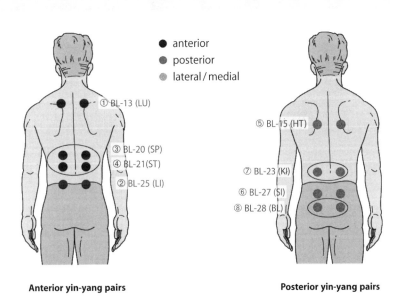

● anterior
● posterior
● lateral / medial

① BL-13 (LU)
③ BL-20 (SP)
④ BL-21(ST)
② BL-25 (LI)

⑤ BL-15 (HT)
⑦ BL-23 (KI)
⑥ BL-27 (SI)
⑧ BL-28 (BL)

Anterior yin-yang pairs

Posterior yin-yang pairs

ASSOCIATED POINTS OF YIN-YANG PAIRS

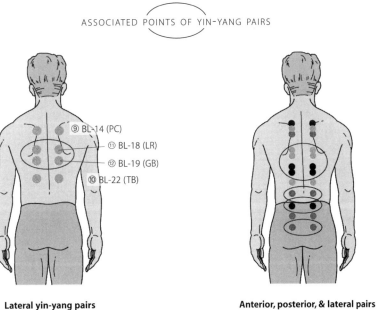

⑨ BL-14 (PC)
⑪ BL-18 (LR)
⑫ BL-19 (GB)
⑩ BL-22 (TB)

Lateral yin-yang pairs

Anterior, posterior, & lateral pairs

Meridian Test Findings Chart

Circle when the movement causes pain, tension, or fatigue (a positive sign) in the stretched part, or on the other side or areas.

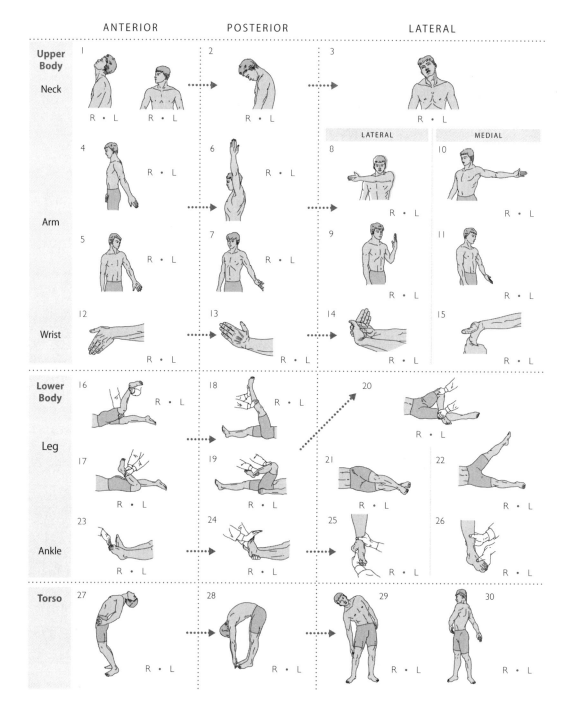

INDEX

Items appearing in figures are marked in **bold**.